LOW-FAT, HIGH-FIBER DIET FOOD PLAN

Super Easy Homemade Recipes to Shed Excess Fat, Prevent Disease, Stroke, Improve Digestion, and Lower High Blood Pressure

Marian Elbert, RDN

Copyright Page

Table of Contents

PART I: UNDERSTANDING LOW-FAT AND HIGH-FIBER DIETS

There are so many different dietary theories out there, where do you even begin? Low-carb, carb-free, vegetarian, vegan, pescatarian, low-FODMAP – the list is seemingly endless. One you may not have considered is a low-fat, high-fiber diet. Many of us are currently (and likely unknowingly) consuming more fat and less fiber than recommended by dietary guidelines.

Fat

Fat is a macronutrient, helping to keep you feeling satisfied after eating, supporting the absorption of fat-soluble vitamins, and contributing to brain development and overall health. There are four types of fats found in food: monounsaturated fats, polyunsaturated fats, saturated fats, and trans fats.

• **Monounsaturated fats** are heart healthy and can be found in nuts, seeds, avocados, and olive oil.

• **Polyunsaturated fats** include the omega-3 and omega-6 fatty acids required in the diet. Sources of polyunsaturated fats include fatty fish, nuts, seeds, and soy.

• **Saturated fats** come from animal-derived foods and tropical oils, and because they're associated with heart disease and weight gain, it's recommended that they be limited in your diet. Unlike mono- and polyunsaturated fats, saturated fats are generally solid at room temperature.

• **Trans fats** are recommended to be avoided completely, as they are inflammatory and linked to heart disease. Trans fats can be found in fried and processed foods.

A low-fat diet is not one that eliminates fat altogether. Instead, it emphasizes low-fat foods and increased awareness of fat sources, with the goal of working toward smaller portions of fatty foods. This type of diet can also help you if your goals include maintaining or losing weight. A successful low-fat diet prioritizes whole, plant-based foods that are naturally lower in fat, especially compared to animal-based foods that contain saturated fats and processed foods that may contain trans fats.

Fiber

Fiber is a type of carbohydrate that cannot be broken down and digested. It comes in two forms, soluble fiber and insoluble fiber, and boasts many health benefits, including keeping your bowel movements regular, lowering your cholesterol and blood pressure, decreasing your risk of developing heart disease and some cancers, controlling blood sugar levels, and maintaining your weight.

The Mayo Clinic's daily fiber recommendations for adults are:

• Men 50 and under: 38 grams

• Women 50 and under: 25 grams

• Men 51 and over: 30 grams

• Women 51 and over: 21 grams

Many people are not meeting these daily recommendations, but it can be simple to do! One of the simplest ways to increase your fiber intake is to eat more whole plant sources of fiber, like legumes, fruits and vegetables, and whole grains.

You may want to take it slow when staring to incorporate more fiber-rich foods into your diet, to avoid digestive discomfort. Be sure to drink plenty of water as you increase your fiber consumption in order to help keep things moving along through the digestive tract.

Importance of dietary fats and fibers for health

Researchers have documented several benefits of dietary fiber. Although more research is necessary on this topic, a 2020 review of the scientific research details the following possible outcomes of high fiber diets:

• prevention or treatment of constipation

• weight loss

• maintenance of health metabolism

• improvement in gut bacteria health

• reduced inflammation

- decreased risk of depression

- improved life expectancy

- colorectal cancer prevention

Dietary fats are essential to give your body energy and to support cell growth. They also help protect your organs and help keep your body warm. Fats help your body absorb some nutrients and produce important hormones, too. Eating moderate amounts of food high in unsaturated fat can help lower your risk of heart disease or stroke, raise good cholesterol while lowering bad cholesterol in your blood, maintain your body's cells and brain health, enhance absorption of certain vitamins, fight inflammation, and reduce your risk of premature death.

How dietary choices impact overall well-being

1. Your Heart Health Improves

The World Health Organization (WHO) estimates over one-third of deaths worldwide are caused by heart disease — and most of those deaths are preventable with lifestyle modifications, especially a well-balanced diet.

You see, a diet high in saturated fats, refined carbs and added sugar lead to the factors that put you at risk for CVD, such as hypertension, type 2 diabetes and obesity. Heart disease is not a disease that sneaks up on your body — it takes years to develop, and you just have to pay attention to signs.

One of the first signs is blood pressure that slowly creeps up. A healthy blood pressure reading is defined as one that's under 120/80, according to the American Heart Association (AHA). While genetics and age definitely play a role in your blood pressure, you aren't destined to have high levels.

A well-balanced diet is naturally low in salt. (Most of the sodium in an unhealthy diet comes from highly processed foods, like hot dogs, deli meat, chicken nuggets and french fries.) In fact, over a period of five years, researchers found that people with a higher intake of ultra-processed foods had a higher risk of developing heart disease, according to a May 2019 study in The BMJ.

When you eat healthier foods, those risk factors naturally decrease. For example, adding more fruits and vegetables to your diet naturally gives you more potassium. Potassium pulls sodium out of your body, which helps lower your blood pressure.

There are other ways healthy eating benefits your heart. Taking in less saturated fat, for example, can significantly lower your risk of heart disease, according to the American Heart Association.

Limit saturated fat to 10 percent or less of your total daily calories (this amounts to about 22 grams per 2,000 calories), per the USDA Dietary Guidelines for Americans.

As far as fat is concerned, you'll want to steer clear of trans fats. They are officially banned in the U.S., but that doesn't mean to you still won't find them in your foods. Anything that says "hydrogenated" or "partially hydrogenated" in the ingredient list means it contains trans fat.

Even if 2 percent of your diet is made up from trans fat, your risk for heart disease can jump 23 percent, according to Harvard Health Publishing.

2. Your Gut Flourishes

If thinking about the bacteria in your gut creeps you out, just imagine them as little helpers working to keep you healthy. Gut health has been implicated in conditions like obesity and type 2 diabetes, as well as your immune health.

When it comes to the gut, a diverse array of bacteria, as these bacteria play different roles in supporting your health. There are many factors that can reduce diversity in your gut (such as use of antibiotics and laxatives, or smoking), but one way you can support it is through your diet.

Some foods that decrease the diversity in your gut include sugar-sweetened beverages, bread and savory snacks, according to July 2019 research in Nutrients. Foods that increase beneficial bacteria in your gut include prebiotics and dietary fiber.

Prebiotics are fermented by the bacteria in the gut, which helps them grow and diversify. Examples of prebiotic foods are green bananas, onions, garlic and apples. These are all sources of fiber as well, and increasing the fiber in your diet is good for your gut.

One noticeable change to your gut health after you add healthy foods is a decrease in bloating. If your current diet is filled with salty, processed foods, you may be carrying around a little extra water, which can cause your belly to distend.

Replacing those salty foods with fresh, whole foods may help flush that salt out of your body and banish the bloat.

3. Your Skin May Improve

The link between diet and skin health is still not completely understood. But what we do know is that changes in nutrition can affect the structure and function of skin, according to the Linus Pauling Institute.

Collagen is a protein that gives skin elasticity, and collagen formation decreases as you age, according to August 2017 research on Nutrients. Vitamin C helps with collagen formation, and some studies have shown that increasing vitamin C in the diet boosts skin elasticity, so that's good news.

Sun damage is also bad for the skin and vitamin C helps protect the skin against UV exposure. Another clearly established role of vitamin C in skin health is that it aids wound healing.

All of these benefits make a good case for eating more foods high in vitamin C. Getting the recommended daily amount of five servings of fruits and vegetables per day will do it.

Just one-half cup of red bell pepper will give you over 100 percent of the daily value of vitamin C, per the USDA. More vitamin C powerhouses are kiwi, strawberries, oranges and broccoli.

4. You Might Lose Weight

One of the most (if not the most) important factors in weight management is diet. If you have overweight or obesity, adopting a nutritious eating pattern can help.

But it's not all about reducing calories: Changing your diet so that you're prioritizing foods that provide adequate macronutrients (carbs, fat and protein) may be more beneficial for weight loss and maintenance, according to June 2017 research in Perspectives on Psychological Science

.

Eating more fruits, vegetables and low-fat dairy has been linked to weight loss as well as weight maintenance, per a

December 2011 review in the Journal of the Academy of Nutrition and Dietetics.

When you make healthier choices in your diet, your weight will most likely be the first thing you notice dropping. There are many types of diets you could follow, but one of the best ones is the Mediterranean diet — it has been ranked number one by the U.S. News and World Report for four years in a row.

Mediterranean diet recipes focus on plant-based foods such as fruits, vegetables, whole grains, beans and nuts — all key components of weight loss and maintenance.

Those who follow this diet pattern eat more lean poultry and fish than red meat and also use olive oil as their fat of choice. Making these changes may help you lose weight by focusing on healthier food choices.

5. You Could Get Stronger

After a certain age, your body doesn't repair and build muscle mass the same way that it used to. This can make your muscles weaker, which puts you at a higher risk of injury, and can also zap your energy levels.

Eating enough protein, especially if you're over 30, can help you prevent the muscle loss that naturally occurs with aging, according to Harvard Health Publishing. Including lean proteins at every meal supports your body in repairing and growing muscle tissue, which in time, may help you feel stronger and more energized.

Both animal sources — poultry, beef, fish, dairy and eggs — as well as plant sources, such as beans, nuts, lentils and soy, are great ways to incorporate more protein into your diet.

6. Your Mental Health May Improve

It may come as no surprise, but your food affects your mood in a pretty significant way. These days, nutrition therapy is often used in combination with other modalities to help with depression.

In fact, low levels of omega-3 fatty acids, vitamin B12, folate (vitamnn B9) and vitamin D were all linked with higher incidences of depression, per a September 2019 review in Antioxidants.

These nutrients, and others such as iron, vitamin A, vitamin C and zinc, were found to have antidepressant properties, per a September 2018 study in the World Journal of Psychiatry.

According to the Mental Health Foundation, making the following diet changes can stabilize your energy levels, support your brain health and help regulate your mood.

Eating regularly to prevent blood sugar drops

Staying hydrated

Focusing on whole grains, fruits and vegetables

Eating protein at every meal

Minding your gut health

Reducing caffeine

7. Your Brain Fog May Subside

The way you eat has a huge influence on your ability to think clearly and remember things (and not just where you put your car keys).

The Mediterranean diet and the DASH (dietary approaches to stop hypertension) diet, two widely-studied diets for their positive effects on brain health, are both full of healthy plant-based foods and low in animal fats.

And diets high in fruits and vegetables and low in saturated fat and salt, specifically, have been linked to improved cognitive function, according to May 2019 research in Nutrients.

If brain fog has you walking around in the clouds and unable to focus, you might be deficient in vitamin B12. This nutrient is important for nerve function, which could affect the connections made between nerves and the brain, per Harvard Health Publishing.

You get B12 from foods like meat, eggs, fish and dairy products. As you age, your body doesn't absorb as much B12 from foods, so it's important to get your levels checked. Plus, people on a vegan diet are at greater risk for B12 deficiency.

If your brain fog is caused by a nutrient deficiency, you could see improvements as soon as your body has a healthy amount available. For memory and cognition, the changes may come slower, but the long-term effects of healthy eating on your brain are worth it.

8. You'll Have Balanced Blood Sugar Levels

Reducing added sugars, increasing fiber and eating protein at every meal are just a few of the many ways to help keep your blood sugar under control.

Eating nutritious foods helps with weight control, and that's key to preventing or controlling type 2 diabetes. If you have overweight, losing only 5 to 10 percent of your body weight can help control your blood sugar if you already have type 2 diabetes or pre-diabetes.

If you have pre-diabetes, losing that small percentage of weight is linked to cutting your risk of getting type 2 diabetes by 58 percent, according to Johns Hopkins Medicine. That's a huge incentive to start improving your diet to prevent a chronic illness.

9. Your Social Life May Flourish

Think about it: When you feel better physically, you're more likely to seek out and enjoy social activities. When you're lacking energy or feeling unwell, the opposite may be true, making it harder to develop social relationships in your community.

There's some interesting research on the relationship between healthy eating and social health. For example, eating a nutritious diet was associated with better social behavior and development in children in an April 2017 study in Maternal and Child Nutrition. Kids who ate healthier diets showed more friendliness and social play than kids who didn't.

Our relationships, with others and with ourselves, are both affected by the foods we eat. Eating a nutritious diet can lead to weight loss, increased energy and improved mental health.

Feeling good on the inside can give you more self-confidence or a more positive self-image. Higher self-esteem can make you more confident socially, strengthening your desire to forge new friendships and romantic connections.

Eating well can be a social activity. Creating recipes in the kitchen with your family or sitting down for nutritious, home-cooked meals can serve as bonding rituals that connect you with those you love.

Low-Fat, High-Fiber Foods

If when you think of low-fat and high-fiber foods, you envision boring and brown processed bars or fiber supplements, instead imagine an abundance of colorful plant-forward foods that meet your fiber and other nutrient needs with plenty of flavors.

Many packaged foods are labeled with health and nutrient claims like "low-fat," "reduced-fat," "light," and "fat-free" on food labels, but beware – these items often contain artificial ingredients and additives like sugars, salt, and thickeners to replicate the filling feeling that fats provide.

Remember, fat is a vital macronutrient! Fat is often viewed in a negative light, but this macronutrient is just as essential as protein and carbs. It allows your body to store energy and absorb and transport fat-soluble vitamins, and it fuels your brain – which is almost 60% fat.

1. Beans

Beans are a super-affordable source of plant-based protein and fiber. There are many varieties to choose from; common types include garbanzo beans, black beans, and red and white kidney beans. One cup of garbanzo beans (or chickpeas) contains 12g of fiber, and one cup of cooked kidney beans contains 16g of fiber. Beans make a delicious addition to salads, soups, and stews.

2. Berries

Berries are some of the highest-fiber fruits per serving. In addition, they are naturally low in fat and high in antioxidants, vitamins, and minerals. One cup of raspberries or blackberries has 8g of fiber. Add fresh or frozen berries to your smoothies for a bright, fiber-rich boost!

3. Cruciferous vegetables

It's no secret that cruciferous vegetables are nutrient-dense; this family of fibrous vegetables contains anti-inflammatory phytonutrients. One cup of broccoli has about 2.4g of fiber, while one cup of Brussels sprouts has about 4g of fiber. Cruciferous veggies are easy to roast or steam, and they add color and texture to stir-fries and side dishes.

4. Whole grains

When focusing on fiber, prioritize whole grains that contain their fiber-rich outer layer (called bran). One serving, or one-half cup, of uncooked rolled oats has 4g of fiber. One cup of cooked bulgur has twice that amount, at 8g of fiber. Whole grains serve as an excellent base for breakfasts or grain bowls with endless combinations of toppings.

5. Seeds

Seeds pack a powerful punch for their size. Just one ounce of flaxseed has 8g of fiber, and one ounce of chia seeds has 10g of fiber! Both types of these seeds are also plant-based sources of omega-3 fatty acids. Sprinkle seeds on just about anything for a bit of crunch.

6. Nuts

A small handful of raw nuts that are not heavily seasoned or roasted in added oil can be a great source of monounsaturated fats, antioxidants, and fiber. One ounce of pistachios contains 3g of fiber, and one ounce of almonds contains 4g of fiber. Nuts and nut butters are versatile ingredients that can easily be paired with other high-fiber foods like oats, fruits, and vegetables.

Low-Fat, High-Fiber Meal Ideas

A low-fat, high-fiber diet can be an important part of a weight-loss journey or a way to support overall healthy living. If you're feeling inspired to incorporate more low-fat, high-fiber foods into your diet, consider the following as inspiration for all the different ways you can combine these nutrient-dense foods.

This diet plan is not meant to serve as a diagnosis or treatment for any dietary-related condition. Please seek medical advice from your health care provider to better understand your bio-individual requirements before implementing a change to your diet.

Breakfast ideas

Keep breakfast simple with a nourishing bowl of berry overnight oats. Thanks to this recipe, you'll start your day with healthy complex carbohydrates, fiber, minerals, vitamins, antioxidants from the colorful berries, and healthy fats. If you'd like, feel free to bulk up the fiber content even more, with another handful of mixed berries or the addition of a spoonful of peanut butter!

If you prefer a savory breakfast, try this vegan tofu scramble from Bree's Vegan Life. This recipe is 224 calories per serving, 9g fat, and 6g of fiber. You can customize this scramble by adding whatever vegetables you like. Broccoli florets and some slices of avocado would add extra fiber and healthy fat!

Snack ideas

Some satisfying snacks include an apple with nut butter; a tropical green smoothie; carrots and hummus; edamame dip atop whole-grain crackers; air-popped popcorn; or homemade trail mix with your favorite nuts, seeds, and dried fruits.

PART II: THE SCIENCE BEHIND LOW-FAT DIETS

A low-fat diet is an eating plan that substantially limits the amount of dietary fat consumed, regardless of the type of fat. Those who follow the eating plan may be seeking weight loss, weight maintenance, or other outcomes like improved heart health.

foods included in a low-fat diet may be naturally low in fat or fat-free, like fruits and vegetables. The diet may also include processed foods that are manufactured to contain less fat than their traditional counterparts, like low-fat cookies or low-fat ice cream.

Exploring different types of fats and their effects on health

Saturated Fat

Saturated fats are fats that are solid at room temperature. They are not unhealthy in the appropriate amounts, but too much can lead to potential health problems. The 2020–2025 Dietary Guidelines for Americans from the U.S. Department of Agriculture recommends keeping your daily intake of saturated fat to less than 10% of your total calories.

For someone eating a 2,000-calorie-per-day diet, an appropriate saturated fat intake would be 22 grams or less, which equals 200 calories.

Some experts believe saturated fat leads to high cholesterol levels—especially "bad" LDL cholesterol. This link could mean that saturated fats contribute to heart disease risk. While some studies support the premise that saturated fat raises cholesterol levels, leading to heart disease, others say the opposite. For instance, the saturated fats in dairy may even provide a protective effect.

If you have high cholesterol or your doctor has recommended you cut back on saturated fats, it's best to do so. Keep in mind that 22 grams of saturated fats are a substantial amount and eating below that level should be fairly easy if you follow a low-fat diet or a nutritionally balanced diet.

Trans Fat

Trans fats are also solid at room temperature. Trans fats can raise LDL cholesterol (the "bad" kind) and lower HDL cholesterol, increasing the risk of cardiovascular disease and diabetes. The recommended intake of trans fats is very low, to zero. The American Heart Association recommends less than 1 percent of your daily calories come from trans fats. For a person eating 2,000 calories per day, that's 2 grams of trans fats, which is 18 calories.

Trans fats are most often artificially produced by adding hydrogen to oils to create more double bonds, making the fats more shelf stable. Some animal foods contain trace amounts of naturally occurring trans fat, which is thought to be less damaging to health.

Unsaturated Fat

Unsaturated fats include mono and polyunsaturated varieties which are found in plant and animal foods like nuts, seeds, fish, avocados, and olive oil. Both types remain liquid at room temperature and are considered "good" fats due to their health-promoting benefits, namely, reducing levels of LDL cholesterol. As well, those who consume more unsaturated fats have decreased risk levels for developing cardiovascular disease.

Instead of following a low-fat diet, experts suggest focusing on increasing your amounts of healthy, unsaturated fats and reducing trans fats while limiting saturated ones. The quality of fat you include in your diet is much more significant for your health than the quantity you consume.

How Much Fat Should I Eat?

Experts recommend that most adults get 20%-35% of their daily calories from fat. That's about 44 to 77 grams of fat a day if you eat 2,000 calories a day.

Read nutrition labels on food packages. Nutrition labels show the number of grams of fat per serving and calories per serving. Eat a variety of lower-fat foods to get all the nutrients you need.

Eat mostly plant foods (such as vegetables, fruits, and whole grains) and a moderate amount of lean and low-fat, animal-based food (meat and dairy products) to help control your fat, cholesterol, carbs, and calories.

When you're shopping, choose fish, poultry, and lean meats. Limit these to 5-7 ounces per day.

Other good low-fat sources of protein include dried beans and peas, tofu, low-fat yogurt, low-fat or skim milk, low-fat cheese, and tuna packed in water.

Choose foods rich in omega-3 fatty acids such as salmon, flaxseed, and walnuts for heart health. The American Heart Association recommends eating fatty fish such as salmon twice weekly for the benefits of omega-3 fatty acids.

Benefits of reducing dietary fat intake for heart health and weight management

Limiting your fat intake as a means of calorie control or to improve health does have some benefits.

• **No foods off-limits**: This isn't a highly restrictive diet in that no foods are categorically off-limits. Even foods high in fat can be consumed in smaller amounts as long as your total daily fat intake falls within your goal range.

• **Can be effective**: In comparison with other diets, some studies indicate that a healthy low-fat diet can be effective for weight loss, although diet quality matters significantly and a low-fat diet isn't necessarily more effective than other diets.

• **Promotes nutritious foods**: Fruits and vegetables supply vitamins and minerals, as well as dietary fiber, which is linked to a decreased risk of cardiovascular disease and obesity. Vitamins and minerals are sources of phytochemicals that function as antioxidants, phytoestrogens, and anti-inflammatory agents.

• **Aligns with some dietary guidelines on fat**: The National Heart Lung and Blood Institute recommends choosing part-skim mozzarella cheese instead of whole milk mozzarella and low-fat (1%), reduced-fat (2%), or fat-free (skim) milk instead of full-fat milk.

• **Inexpensive and accessible**: You can choose to go on a low-fat diet without paying for a subscription service or buying special meals. Low-fat foods (both naturally low in fat and manufactured low-fat) are readily available in almost every grocery store.

• **May improve heart health**: If you reduce your intake of saturated fat on a low-fat diet, you may be able to reduce your risk of cardiovascular disease. The American Heart Association suggests consuming no more than 13 grams of saturated fat per day (equal to about 5% or 6% of total daily calories), as this type of fat is linked to a higher risk for heart disease. By watching your fat intake on a low-fat diet, you may become more mindful about healthier fat choices and consume mono- and polyunsaturated fats instead.

• **Reduced risk of cardiovascular disease**: Some studies have shown that men who reduced total fat and saturated fat from 36% and 12% of total calories to 27% and 8% of total calories, respectively, saw a substantial decline in their total and LDL cholesterol levels. Similarly, many studies have linked a reduction in saturated fat intake with a reduced risk for cardiovascular disease.

• **May prevent certain cancers**: Some studies suggest that reducing dietary fat intake may prevent cancers of the breast, colon, rectum, and prostate. But that doesn't necessarily mean that reducing your fat intake below recommended levels is advised.

• **May result in weight loss**: A low-fat diet has been associated with weight loss for decades. While there are anecdotal reports of weight loss on a low-fat diet, and some studies do support the fact that weight loss can occur on a low-fat diet, there is no strong evidence that a low-fat diet is more effective than other diets.

Cons of Low Fat Diets

Nutrition and health experts do have some concerns about low-fat diets. But as with the beneficial aspects of the diet, the nutritional quality of the foods consumed makes a big difference in mitigating potential health risks.

• **Reduces intake of nutrients**: Healthy fats provide key benefits to the body. Your body needs dietary fat to absorb vitamins A, D, E, and K. Fat supports healthy cell growth and protects your body's organs. Healthy fats can also keep cholesterol and blood pressure under control. By severely reducing your fat intake, especially to levels below what is recommended by the USDA, you may limit these benefits, and your body may not get the nutrients it needs.

• **Hard to sustain**: Fat helps you to feel full and provides a satisfying mouthfeel in foods. Without the satiating qualities of fat during meals and snacks, you may end up overeating other foods and increasing your caloric intake, sugar intake, or carb intake to levels that are not consistent with your goals.

• **May increase intake of less healthy foods**: When the low-fat diet first became the diet of choice among Americans, several brands developed ultra-processed, low-fat alternatives to traditionally high-fat foods, like cookies, ice cream, and chips. These foods are often high in sugar or starch and may actually inhibit your health goals rather than help. Many of the foods provide little in the way of good nutrition, and some studies even suggest that overconsuming them may lead to problems with excessive weight gain and diabetes.

• **May result in macronutrient imbalances**: In some cases, going low-fat can lead to a nutritional imbalance. For instance, if you cut back on fat but maintain your caloric intake and protein intake, you're likely to consume more carbohydrates. The USDA suggests that adults consume 45% to 65% of calories from carbs. If you are only

consuming 10% of calories from fat and less than 25% of
your calories from protein, your carb intake will be above
the recommended guidelines.

• **May increase intake of refined carbohydrates**:
Carbohydrate quality matters as well. Some companies make
low-fat foods by replacing fat with large amounts of refined
carbohydrates. Frequently consuming highly processed,
low-fat foods packed with refined carbohydrates may
increase the risk of metabolic disorders and
hypertriglyceridemia.

• **May not be effective for long-term weight loss**: If weight
loss is your goal, going low-fat may not be your best option.
Several studies have compared a low-fat diet to other types
of weight-loss diets (like low-carb diets). In one
comprehensive review published in 2015, researchers found
that higher fat, low-carbohydrate diets led to greater long-
term weight loss than low-fat diets.

May result in micronutrient imbalances: Lastly, you may
not get all of the micronutrients you need if you reduce your
fat intake significantly. Your body needs dietary fat to
absorb vitamins A, D, E, and K. And many fatty foods, like

nuts, seeds, avocado, olives, and dairy products, are good sources of nutrients like fiber, protein, and calcium

Foods to Include and Avoid

What You Can Eat

There is no single specific way to follow a low-fat diet. Many popular and commercial diet plans are low-fat diets but use different approaches to reduce fat intake. For example, some diets use fat-free meal replacement shakes or low-fat frozen meals.

Others encourage cooking and preparing meals without fats like butter or cooking oils. Low-fat diets can be healthy, but some low-fat diets reduce or eliminate foods that provide important nutrients, enjoyment, and satiety.

Fruits and Vegetables

These foods are usually low in fat, except for avocado and olives. In order to get a variety of healthy nutrients on a low-fat diet, it is generally recommended that you consume fruits and vegetables in all colors of the rainbow.

- Apples

- Oranges

- Melons

- Berries

- Carrots

- Leafy greens

- Asparagus

- Potatoes

- Squash

Low-Fat Dairy

Most full-fat dairy products have a lower fat counterpart, and certain low-fat items provide calcium and protein.

- Low-fat or fat-free yogurt

- Low-fat cheese

- Skim milk

- Low-fat cottage cheese

- Low-fat sour cream

Grains, Legumes and Pulses

Grains, legumes, and pulses provide carbohydrates for energy and are a good source of protein for those on a low-fat diet. Meat intake may be reduced on this eating plan, so getting protein from other sources is important.

• Whole grains

• Legumes (beans)

• Pulses (lentils and peas)

• Whole grain bread products

Lean Protein

Many protein sources are low in fat. Choose from these options.

• Skinless poultry

• White fish (cod, halibut)

• Lean cuts of beef (flank steak, filet mignon)

• Lean cuts of pork (pork tenderloin, extra-lean ground pork)

• Egg whites

Low-Fat Sweets

There are many low-fat and fat-free sweets available, but it's important to note that they are likely to be high in sugar. This includes frozen treats like sherbet or sorbet and certain types of candy like licorice or hard candy. While these foods are allowed on a low-fat diet, they don't contribute substantial vitamins or minerals and tend to be high in sugar.

What You Cannot Eat

In general, low-fat diets limit your fat intake to 30% or less of your total daily calorie intake.10 Some low-fat diets restrict fat severely, lower than 15% of caloric intake. The foods listed below are not strictly banned, but would likely be very limited on a low-fat diet in order to stay within caloric limits.

Full-Fat Dairy Products

These foods contribute substantial fat grams.

• Full-fat cheese

• Full fat milk

• Cream

• Full fat sour cream

• Full fat yogurt

High-Fat Sweets

Popular baked treats are usually made with eggs, oil, and butter that are high in fat. These foods are usually eliminated completely or substantially reduced on a low-fat diet.

• Cakes

• Pies

• Cupcakes

• Muffins

• Chocolate bars

Nuts and Seeds

The fats in most nuts and seeds provide good fat, but they are generally avoided because they are higher in fat. However, when consuming a low-fat diet, you will still want to add small portions of these foods to your diet so that you are getting all of their essential fatty acids. Keep portion size in mind.

• Almonds

• Walnuts

• Chia seeds

• Flaxseed

• Sunflower seeds

Avocado and Olives

These fruits are mostly fat, making them off-limits on a low-fat diet. For instance, an avocado provides 21 grams of fat—which for some people on this diet may be a full day's supply of the nutrient.11

Fatty Meats

Meats that are not very lean are usually eliminated or reduced on a low-fat diet.

• Processed meats and cold cuts

• Medium ground meat

• Well-marbled steak

Oils

Plant-based oils provide healthy fat, and some are even associated with better heart health.12 However, they are used sparingly or not at all on a low-fat diet. Some people on the diet choose to use a cooking spray instead of oil when cooking foods at home to control portions.

• Canola oil

• Olive oil

• Sunflower oil

• Coconut oil

• Butter

Sample Shopping List

You'll find many low-fat foods (both processed and naturally low in fat) in most grocery stores. To keep your low-fat eating plan healthy, try to spend most of your time in the outer aisles of the store, like the produce section. In the dairy aisle, look for low-fat alternatives and be prepared to read nutritional labels on packaged foods (like cereals, condiments, and grains) in the inner aisles.

Since the low-fat diet is flexible in terms of food choices, this is not a definitive shopping list and if following the diet, you may find other foods that work best for you.

• Fresh fruits and vegetables in a variety of colors (red peppers, oranges, leafy greens, blueberries, eggplant, etc.)

• Frozen fruits or vegetables (often less expensive than fresh, and won't spoil quickly)

• Grains, preferably whole grains such as quinoa, oatmeal, brown rice

• Beans and legumes (black beans, kidney beans, red beans, lentils)

• Low-fat fish (tilapia, cod, sole)

• Lean skinless protein such as chicken or turkey breast

PART III: EMBRACING A HIGH-FIBER LIFESTYLE

Fiber is a macronutrient and a type of carbohydrate found naturally in plant-based foods that is not digestible in humans.

Plant-based foods that are rich in fiber — fruits, vegetables, whole grains, beans and legumes, and nuts and seeds, per the U.S. Department of Agriculture's guidelines — also contain vitamins, minerals, and other powerful nutrients the body can use for optimal health.

Although fiber cannot be digested, it moves down the digestive tract with nutrients as they're digested, and does some great things to positively impact our health along the way.

But fewer than 1 in 10 American adults meet their daily fiber recommendation, according to the American Society for Nutrition.

The appropriate level for most adults is between 22 and 34 grams (g) of fiber per day, depending on age and sex, as the 2020–2025 Dietary Guidelines for Americans state.

Types of Dietary Fiber

Fiber is commonly classified as soluble, which dissolves in water, or insoluble, which doesn't dissolve.

Soluble fiber: This type of fiber dissolves in water to form a gel-like material. It can help lower blood cholesterol and glucose levels. Soluble fiber is found in oats, peas, beans, apples, citrus fruits, carrots, barley and psyllium.

Insoluble fiber: This type of fiber promotes the movement of material through your digestive system and increases stool bulk, so it can be of benefit to those who struggle with constipation or irregular stools. Whole-wheat flour, wheat bran, nuts, beans and vegetables, such as cauliflower, green beans and potatoes, are good sources of insoluble fiber.

The amount of soluble and insoluble fiber varies in different plant foods. To receive the greatest health benefit, eat a wide variety of high-fiber foods.

There is also a lot of overlap between soluble and insoluble fibers. Some insoluble fibers can be digested by the good bacteria in the intestine, and most foods contain both soluble and insoluble fibers.

Health authorities recommend that men and women eat 38 and 25 grams of fiber per day, respectively.

Health benefits of a high-fiber diet, including digestive health and weight control

Fiber feeds "good" gut bacteria

The bacteria that live in the human body outnumber the body's cells 10 to 1. Bacteria live on the skin, in the mouth, and in the nose, but the great majority live in the gut, primarily the large intestine.

Five hundred to 1,000 different species of bacteria live in the intestine, totaling about 38 trillion cells. These gut bacteria are also known as the gut flora.

This is not a bad thing. In fact, there is a mutually beneficial relationship between you and some of the bacteria that live in your digestive system.

You provide food, shelter, and a safe habitat for the bacteria. In return, they take care of some things that the human body cannot do on its own.

Of the many different kinds of bacteria, some are crucial for various aspects of your health, including weight, blood sugar control, immune function, and even brain function.

You may wonder what this has to do with fiber. Just like any other organism, bacteria need to eat to get energy to survive and function.

The problem is that most carbs, proteins, and fats are absorbed into the bloodstream before they make it to the large intestine, leaving little for the gut flora.

This is where fiber comes in. Human cells don't have the enzymes to digest fiber, so it reaches the large intestine relatively unchanged.

However, intestinal bacteria do have the enzymes to digest many of these fibers.

This is the most important reason that (some) dietary fibers are essential for health. They feed the "good" bacteria in the intestine, functioning as prebiotics.

In this way, they promote the growth of "good" gut bacteria, which can have various positive effects on health.

The friendly bacteria produce nutrients for the body, including short-chain fatty acids such as acetate, propionate, and butyrate, of which butyrate appears to be the most important.

These short-chain fatty acids can feed the cells in the colon, leading to reduced gut inflammation and improvements in digestive disorders such as irritable bowel syndrome, Crohn's disease, and ulcerative colitis.

When the bacteria ferment the fiber, they also produce gases. This is why high fiber diets can cause flatulence and stomach discomfort in some people. These side effects usually go away with time as your body adjusts.

Lower Odds of Heart Disease

According to a 2022 BMC Public Health study, a higher fiber intake was associated with a reduced risk for cardiovascular disease (CVD) in a large group of Americans. Researchers don't completely understand how fiber works, but they think that soluble fiber plays a role in decreasing lipid uptake from the intestinal tract, resulting in lower blood levels of cholesterol according to a 2023 Advances in Nutrition review. In addition, experts say that dietary fiber reduces inflammation which can result in CVD in a 2022 JAMA Network Open article.

Some types of fiber can help you lose weight

Certain types of fiber can help you lose weight by reducing your appetite.

In fact, some studies show that increasing dietary fiber can cause weight loss by automatically reducing calorie intake.

Fiber can soak up water in the intestine, slowing the absorption of nutrients and increasing feelings of fullness.

However, this depends on the type of fiber. Some types have no effect on weight, while certain soluble fibers can have a significant effect.

A good example of an effective fiber supplement for weight loss is glucomannan.

Fiber can reduce blood sugar spikes after a high carb meal

High fiber foods tend to have a lower glycemic index than refined carb sources, which have been stripped of most of their fiber.

However, scientists believe that only high viscosity, soluble fibers have this property.

Including these viscous, soluble fibers in your carb-containing meals may cause smaller spikes in blood sugar.

This is important, especially if you're following a high carb diet. In this case, the fiber can reduce the likelihood of the carbs raising your blood sugar to harmful levels.

That said, if you have blood sugar issues, you should consider reducing your carb intake — especially your intake of low fiber, refined carbs such as white flour and added sugar.

Fiber can reduce cholesterol, but the effect isn't huge

Viscous, soluble fiber can also reduce your cholesterol levels.

However, the effect isn't nearly as impressive as you might expect.

A review of 67 controlled studies found that consuming 2–10 grams of soluble fiber per day reduced total cholesterol by only 1.7 mg/dl and LDL (bad) cholesterol by 2.2 mg/dl, on average.

But this also depends on the viscosity of the fiber. Some studies have found impressive reductions in cholesterol with increased fiber intake.

Whether this has any meaningful effects in the long term is unknown, although many observational studies show that people who eat more fiber have a lower risk of heart disease.

Fiber might reduce the risk of colorectal cancer

Colorectal cancer is the third leading cause of cancer deaths in the world.

Many studies have linked a high intake of fiber-rich foods with a reduced risk of colon cancer.

However, whole, high fiber foods like fruits, vegetables, and whole grains contain various other healthy nutrients and antioxidants that may affect cancer risk.

Therefore, it's difficult to isolate the effects of fiber from other factors in healthy, whole-food diets. To date, no strong evidence proves that fiber has cancer-preventive effects.

Yet, since fiber may help keep the colon wall healthy, many scientists believe that fiber plays an important role.

More Regular Bowel Movements

One of the main benefits of increasing fiber intake is reduced constipation.

Fiber is believed to help absorb water, increase the bulk of stool, and speed up the movement of stool through the intestine. However, the evidence is fairly conflicting.

Longer Life

A 2022 review in the Journal of Translational Medicine found that people who ate enough total fiber—which includes soluble and insoluble fibers—had a lower chance of dying early from anything, including cardiovascular disease and cancer. This means that even if you were to get heart disease, cancer or another condition, consuming enough fiber may protect you from dying from it.

Some studies show that increasing fiber can improve symptoms of constipation, but other studies show that removing fiber improves constipation. The effects depend on the type of fiber.

In one study in 63 individuals with chronic constipation, going on a low fiber diet fixed their problem. The individuals who remained on a high fiber diet saw no improvement.

In general, fiber that increases the water content of your stool has a laxative effect, while fiber that adds to the dry mass of stool without increasing its water content may have a constipating effect.

Soluble fibers that form a gel in the digestive tract and are not fermented by gut bacteria are often effective. A good example of a gel-forming fiber is psyllium.

Other types of fiber, such as sorbitol, have a laxative effect by drawing water into the colon. Prunes are a good source of sorbitol.

Choosing the right type of fiber may help your constipation, but taking the wrong supplements can do the opposite.

For this reason, you should consult a healthcare professional before taking fiber supplements for constipation.

All-Natural Detox

Fiber naturally scrubs and promotes the elimination of toxins from your GI tract. Soluble fiber soaks up potentially harmful compounds, such as excess estrogen and unhealthy fats, before they can be absorbed by the body. And because insoluble fiber makes things move along more quickly, it limits the amount of time that chemicals like BPA, mercury and pesticides stay in your system. The faster they go through you, the less chance they have to cause harm.

Strong Bones

Some types of soluble fiber—known as prebiotics—have been shown to contribute to a greater bioavailability of minerals, like calcium, in your colon. The increase in bioavailability supports maintain bone density, according to a 2018 review in the journal Calcified Tissue International. Prebiotics provide food for your beneficial gut bacteria and can be found in certain fruits, vegetables, nuts and whole grains, such as asparagus, bananas, walnuts, onions, legumes, wheat and oats.

Foods rich in fiber and how to incorporate them into a daily diet

What foods are most high in fiber?

You've probably already been eating foods that are high in fiber. But just in case — here are a few of our top picks for high fiber foods to add to your plate.

Lentils

20.5 grams of fiber per cup, uncooked

10.7 grams of fiber in every 100 grams

Lentils are a great source of nutrients and an even better source of dietary fiber. Just 1 cup of uncooked lentils nets over 20 grams of fiber, which makes them great for batch recipes like curries, stews, and soups.

Oats

16.5 grams of fiber per cup, uncooked

10.6 grams of fiber in every 100 grams

Oats are another quick, easy, and affordable source of dietary fiber, especially for breakfast. But even if you're not a fan of oats in the morning, you can still use them in other baking recipes, like breads, muffins, and more.

Black beans

15 grams of fiber per cup, cooked

8.7 grams of fiber in every 100 grams

Black beans are a staple in plant-based diets because they're not just high in fiber — they're also a great source of protein. One cup of cooked black beans has 15 grams of fiber, which is around half the recommended daily amount.

Kidney beans

13.1 grams of fiber per cup, cooked

7.4 grams of fiber in every 100 grams

Like black beans, kidney beans are also high in vitamins, minerals, protein, and fiber. Kidney beans are versatile and can be found in a variety of recipes, like vegetarian chili, red beans and rice, and even cold salads.

Chickpeas

12.5 grams of fiber per cup, cooked

7.6 grams of fiber in every 100 grams

Chickpeas are another great plant-based source of protein and dietary fiber. And you might be surprised by all the ways you can eat them — in soups, stews, salads, curries, and even roasted in the oven for a crunchy snack.

Avocado

10 grams of fiber per cup

6.7 grams of fiber in every 100 grams

Avocados are deliciously creamy and nutrient-dense — with plenty of fiber, too. Most people enjoy avocados on toast or in salads, but if you're looking for a little extra fiber in the morning, they also taste great in smoothies.

Chia seeds

9.75 grams of fiber per ounce, dried

34.4 grams of fiber in every 100 grams

Chia seeds are one of the best sources of soluble fiber, the type of fiber that helps slow down digestion and balance blood sugar. If you want to add chia seeds to your diet, your body will process them easier if you soak them first.

Raspberries

8 grams of fiber per cup

6.5 grams of fiber in every 100 grams

Raspberries may seem like a sweet treat, but did you know that they're also high in fiber? Adding 1 cup of these berries to your breakfast or a snack will net you 8 grams of fiber, getting you that much closer to your fiber goal.

Strategies for increasing fiber intake without feeling deprived

Below are tips for fitting in more fiber:

Jump-start your day

For breakfast choose a high-fiber breakfast cereal — 5 or more grams of fiber a serving. Opt for cereals with "whole grain," "bran" or "fiber" in the name. Or add a few tablespoons of unprocessed wheat bran to your favorite cereal.

Switch to whole grains

Consume at least half of all grains as whole grains. Look for breads that list whole wheat, whole-wheat flour or another whole grain as the first ingredient on the label and have at least 2 grams of dietary fiber a serving. Experiment with brown rice, wild rice, barley, whole-wheat pasta and bulgur wheat.

Bulk up baked goods

Substitute whole-grain flour for half or all of the white flour when baking. Try adding crushed bran cereal, unprocessed wheat bran or uncooked oatmeal to muffins, cakes and cookies.

Lean on legumes

Beans, peas and lentils are excellent sources of fiber. Add kidney beans to canned soup or a green salad. Or make nachos with refried black beans, lots of fresh veggies, whole-wheat tortilla chips and salsa.

Eat more fruit and vegetables

Fruits and vegetables are rich in fiber, as well as vitamins and minerals. Try to eat five or more servings daily.

Make snacks count

Fresh fruits, raw vegetables, low-fat popcorn and whole-grain crackers are all good choices. A handful of nuts or dried fruits also is a healthy, high-fiber snack — although be aware that nuts and dried fruits are high in calories.

High-fiber foods are good for your health. But adding too much fiber too quickly can promote intestinal gas, abdominal bloating and cramping. Increase fiber in your diet gradually over a few weeks. This allows the natural bacteria in your digestive system to adjust to the change.

Also, drink plenty of water. Fiber works best when it absorbs water, making your stool soft and bulky.

PART IV: HIGH FIBER, LOW FAT DIET CULINARY CREATIONS AND RECIPES

TASTY HIGH FIBRE DIET RECIPES

TASTY HIGH FIBRE BREAKFAST RECIPES

Staffordshire oatcakes with mushrooms

Ingredients

For the oatcakes

85g porridge oats

85g plain wholemeal flour

½ tsp dried yeast

For the topping

4 tsp rapeseed oil, plus a little for frying

320g button mushrooms, sliced

4 tomatoes, each cut into 8 wedges

4 tbsp milled seeds with flax and chia

4 tbsp tahini

a few coriander sprigs, chopped

Directions

STEP 1

For the oatcakes, tip the oats and 350ml water into a bowl
and blitz with a stick blender until smooth (alternatively you
can use a food processor or liquidizer). Stir in the flour and
yeast, cover and leave in the fridge overnight, or leave at
room temperature for 2-3 hrs until bubbles appear.

STEP 2

Use kitchen paper to rub ½ tsp oil round a non-stick frying
pan, then heat. Ladle in a quarter of the batter and swirl the
pan to cover the base (the oatcakes should be a few

millimeters thick, like a crêpe). Cook for 2 mins, then turn and cook for 2 mins more until golden. Make four oatcakes in the same way. If you're following our Healthy Diet Plan, chill two for another day. Will keep, covered in the fridge, for two days.

STEP 3

To make the topping for two oatcakes, heat 2 tsp oil in a non-stick pan, add 160g mushrooms and fry for 2-3 mins, stirring until softened. Stir in 2 tomatoes, then add 2 tbsp ground seeds and cook for 2 mins more. Reheat the oatcakes in a dry frying pan or the microwave if necessary, then spread each one with 1 tbsp tahini, the mushroom mixture and scatter with a little coriander before serving. On the second day, repeat step 3 with the remaining Ingredients.

Sweetcorn pancakes

Ingredients

a whole corn on the cob or a 330g can of sweetcorn, drained

2medium eggs

5 tbsp milk

25g butter, melted

85g self-raising flour

2 spring onions, finely chopped

4 tbsp sunflower oil, for shallow frying

To serve

4 tomatoes, cut in half

olive oil, for drizzling

8rashers good quality bacon, streaky or back

chilli sauce to serve

Directions

STEP 1

First turn the grill on high. If using fresh corn, remove the husk and slice the kernels from the cob with a large sharp knife, then cook them in a pan of boiling water for 5 minutes. Drain and leave to cool while you whisk the eggs, milk and butter together. Whisk in the flour and a large pinch of salt until smooth, then mix in the corn (fresh or canned) and the spring onions.

STEP 2

Put the tomatoes cut-side up on a large baking tray, drizzle with olive oil and season with salt and pepper. Lay the bacon next to the tomatoes in a single file on the tray. Grill for 8–10 minutes until the tomatoes have softened and the bacon is crispy, turning the rashers over at half time.

STEP 3

While the bacon's crisping up, heat the sunflower oil in a large frying pan. Add 4 large spoonfuls of the batter and fry for 1-2 minutes on each side until the pancakes are puffed up and golden. Lift out on to a plate lined with kitchen paper and cook the remaining 4 pancakes. Bring to the table with a bottle of chilli sauce.

Banana overnight oats

Ingredients

2 bananas, peeled

100g porridge oats

¼ tsp ground cinnamon, plus a pinch to serve

1 tbsp maple syrup

300ml milk of your choice, plus a splash

2 tbsp peanut or almond butter, plus extra to serve

2 tbsp flaked or chopped almonds

2-4 tbsp natural yogurt, to serve (optional)

Directions

STEP 1

Mash 1 banana in a bowl with a fork until smooth. Stir in the oats, cinnamon, maple syrup, milk and peanut butter. Mix well, then cover and chill overnight.

STEP 2

The next morning, stir the porridge, adding another splash of milk if the mixture is quite stiff. Divide between two bowls. Slice the remaining banana and scatter this over the porridge, drizzle with more nut butter and sprinkle over the almonds.

Top with spoonfuls of yogurt, if using, and sprinkle with a pinch more cinnamon before serving.

Peanut Butter & Chocolate Banana Smoothie

Ingredients

1 cup nonfat milk

1 frozen medium banana

2 tablespoons natural peanut butter

1 tablespoon unsweetened cocoa powder

1 tablespoon chia or hemp seeds (optional)

1 teaspoon vanilla extract

Directions

Combine milk, banana, peanut butter, cocoa, chia or hemp seeds (if using) and vanilla in a blender. Puree until smooth

"Egg in a Hole" Peppers with Avocado Salsa

2 bell peppers, any color

1 avocado, diced

½ cup diced red onion

1 jalapeño pepper, minced

½ cup chopped fresh cilantro, plus more for garnish

2 tomatoes, seeded and diced

Juice of 1 lime

¾ teaspoon salt, divided

2 teaspoons olive oil, divided

8 large eggs

¼ teaspoon ground pepper, divided

Directions

1. Slice tops and bottoms off bell peppers and finely dice. Remove and discard seeds and membranes. Slice each pepper into four 1/2-inch-thick rings.

2. Combine the diced pepper with avocado, onion, jalapeño, cilantro, tomatoes, lime juice, and 1/2 teaspoon salt in a medium bowl.

3. Heat 1 teaspoon oil in a large nonstick skillet over medium heat. Add 4 bell pepper rings, then crack 1 egg into the middle of each ring. Season with 1/8 teaspoon each salt and pepper. Cook until the whites are mostly set but the yolks are still runny, 2 to 3 minutes. Gently flip and cook 1 minute more for runny yolks, 1 1/2 to 2 minutes more for firmer yolks. Transfer to serving plates and repeat with the remaining pepper rings and eggs.

4. Serve with the avocado salsa and garnish with additional cilantro, if desired.

Egg Sandwiches with Rosemary, Tomato & Feta

Ingredients

4 multigrain sandwich thins

4 teaspoons olive oil

1 tablespoon snipped fresh rosemary or 1/2 teaspoon dried rosemary, crushed

4 eggs

2 cups fresh baby spinach leaves

1 medium tomato, cut into 8 thin slices

4 tablespoons reduced-fat feta cheese

⅛ teaspoon kosher salt

Freshly ground black pepper

Directions

1. Preheat oven to 375°F. Split sandwich thins; brush cut sides with 2 teaspoons of the olive oil. Place on rimmed baking sheet; toast in oven

2. Meanwhile, in a large skillet heat the remaining 2 teaspoons olive oil and the rosemary over medium-high heat. Break eggs, one at a time, into skillet. Cook about 1 minute or until whites are set but yolks are still runny. Break yolks with spatula. Flip eggs; cook on the other side until done. Remove from heat.

3. Place the bottom halves of the toasted sandwich thins on 4 serving plates. Divide spinach among sandwich thins on plates. Top each with 2 of the tomato slices, an egg and 1 tablespoon of the feta cheese. Sprinkle with the salt

and pepper. Top with the remaining sandwich thin halves.

Tomato-Parmesan Mini Quiches

Ingredients

Nonstick cooking spray

12 4-inch round thin slices lower sodium cooked ham (see Tip)

1 ¼ cups seeded and chopped roma tomatoes

½ cup thinly sliced green onions

1 tablespoon snipped fresh basil or 1 tsp. dried basil, crushed

¼ teaspoon black pepper

⅔ cup finely shredded Parmesan cheese

6 eggs, lightly beaten

Directions

1. Preheat oven to 350 degrees F. Coat twelve 2 1/2-inch muffin cups with cooking spray.

2. Line prepared muffin cups with ham. Divide tomatoes, green onions, basil and pepper among cups. Top with cheese. Pour eggs over tomato mixture.

3. Bake 20 to 25 minutes or until puffed and a knife comes out clean. Cool in cups 5 minutes. Remove from cups. If desired, top with additional green onions and/or fresh basil. Serve warm.

TASTY HIGH FIBRE LUNCH RECIPES

Tuna, spring onion & sweetcorn fritters

Ingredients

125ml milk

3 eggs, beaten

150g self-raising flour

300g frozen sweetcorn, defrosted (or use cooked fresh corn)

½ bunch of spring onions, trimmed and thinly sliced

1 lemon, zested and cut into wedges

2 x 112g cans tuna, drained and roughly flaked

sunflower or vegetable oil, for frying

To serve

100g soured cream

hot sauce, to serve (optional)

Directions

STEP 1

Mix the milk and eggs together in a jug with ½ tsp salt and ¼ tsp ground black pepper. Sift the flour into a bowl, make a well in the centre and pour in the egg mixture in a thin, steady stream, whisking well until combined. Stir in the sweetcorn, spring onions, lemon zest and tuna.

STEP 2

Heat a drop of oil in a non-stick or cast iron frying pan over a medium heat. Drop spoonfuls of the batter into the pan and cook until crisp and golden, about 2-3 mins, flip and repeat on the other side (you'll need to do this in batches). Keep warm in a low oven and repeat with the remaining batter.

Spiced lentil & butternut squash soup

Ingredients

2 tbsp olive oil

2 onions, finely chopped

2 garlic cloves, crushed

¼ tsp hot chilli powder

1 tbsp ras el hanout

1 butternut squash, peeled and cut into 2cm pieces

100g red lentils

1l hot vegetable stock

1 small bunch coriander, leaves chopped, plus extra to serve

dukkah (see tip) and natural yogurt, to serve

Directions

STEP 1

Heat the oil in a large flameproof casserole dish or saucepan over a medium-high heat. Fry the onions with a pinch of salt for 7 mins, or until softened and just caramelised. Add the garlic, chilli and ras el hanout, and cook for 1 min more.

STEP 2

Stir in the squash and lentils. Pour over the stock and season to taste. Bring to the boil, then reduce the heat to a simmer and cook, covered, for 25 mins or until the squash is soft. Blitz the soup with a stick blender until smooth, then season to taste. To freeze, leave to cool completely and transfer to large freezerproof bags.

STEP 3

Stir in the coriander leaves and ladle the soup into bowls. Serve topped with the dukkah, yogurt and extra coriander leaves.

Leek & broccoli soup with cheesy scones

Ingredients

375g leeks, thinly sliced

400g potatoes, peeled and cut into medium chunks

2 garlic cloves, chopped

2 tsp vegetable bouillon powder

340g broccoli, roughly chopped

250ml milk

For the cheese scones

165g plain wholemeal flour

1 tsp baking powder

20g parmesan or vegetarian alternative, finely grated

1 tsp mustard powder

100ml milk

½ tbsp olive oil

65g soft goat's cheese

4 tomatoes, sliced, to serve

Directions

STEP 1

Tip the leeks, potatoes and garlic into a large pan with the bouillon. Pour over 800ml boiling water, stir well, cover and simmer for 15 mins.

STEP 2

Add the broccoli to the pan, then cover and cook for 5 mins more until just tender. Blitz with a hand blender until smooth, then pour in the milk and blitz again. Add a little stock if the soup looks too thick.

STEP 3

To make the scones, heat the oven to 220C/200C fan/gas 7 and line a baking tray with baking parchment. Put the flour and baking powder in a bowl with the all but 1 tbsp of the parmesan and all the mustard powder. Gradually add the milk and oil, stirring with a cutlery knife until the mixture comes together. Shape into a log, about 16cm long and 6cm wide, and press the remaining parmesan on top. Cut in half along the length, then halve each of those pieces again to create four wedge-like scones. Arrange the scones on the tray and bake for 10-12 mins until golden.

Ponzu tofu poke bowl

Ingredients

1 tbsp ponzu sauce

½ tbsp rice vinegar

5g ginger, peeled and grated

1 tsp sesame oil

300g silken tofu

100g edamame beans

250g pouch cooked quinoa

100g radishes, sliced

2 carrots, peeled into ribbons

2 spring onions, finely sliced

2 small seaweed thins, crumbled

1 tsp sesame seeds

Instructions

STEP 1

Combine the ponzu, vinegar, ginger and sesame oil in a bowl. Pat the tofu dry using kitchen paper and tear into chunks, then gently toss in the ponzu mixture.

STEP 2

Pour some boiling water over the edamame and set aside for 2 mins before draining thoroughly and seasoning with salt.

STEP 3

Divide the quinoa between bowls and top with the edamame, radishes and carrots. Spoon over the tofu and drizzle over the remaining dressing before scattering over the spring onions, seaweed and sesame seeds.

Vegan carbonara

Ingredients

360g wholewheat spaghetti

85g unsalted cashew nuts

2 tsp bouillon powder

2 tsp English mustard powder

1 tsp olive oil

200g baby chestnut mushrooms, halved and thinly sliced

3 garlic cloves, 2 finely grated

1 tsp smoked paprika

2 courgettes (about 320g), peeled then grated

4 tsp nutritional yeast flakes, optional

320g spinach, half cooked each evening as a side dish

Instructions

STEP 1

Boil the spaghetti for 10 mins or following pack instructions until al dente, reserving a little of the water. Put the cashews, bouillon and mustard in a bowl, then pour over 350ml boiling water.

STEP 2

Heat the oil in a large non-stick pan. Add the mushrooms and grated garlic, and stir-fry over a high heat until the mushrooms are cooked and starting to crisp up. Take off the heat, stir in the paprika, then tip onto a plate and set aside.

STEP 3

Add the grated courgette to the pan and cook, stirring every now and then until softened. Meanwhile, whizz the soaked cashews, whole garlic clove and nutritional yeast flakes, if using, with a hand blender until completely smooth. Tip the mixture into the pan with the courgettes and briefly stir over the heat.

STEP 4

Add the spaghetti and toss in the cashew and courgette mixture until well coated, then toss through the smoky mushrooms. Serve half with half the spinach on the side, and chill the rest for another day. Will keep for three days. Reheat in a covered pan with a dash of water, and cook the remaining spinach to serve on the side.

Golden noodle soup with soft-boiled eggs

Ingredients

4 medium eggs

400g egg noodles

2 tbsp vegetable oil

2 large garlic cloves, crushed

1 tbsp ginger purée

2 tsp turmeric

400ml low-salt stock, made with 1 low-salt chicken stock cube or 1 tbsp concentrated low-salt liquid stock

2 x 400g cans reduced-fat coconut milk

3 tbsp reduced-salt light soy sauce

1 tbsp light brown soft sugar

150g sugar snap peas

small bunch of spring onions

small handful of coriander leaves

Equipment

small saucepan

slotted spoon

medium-sized saucepan

colander

measuring spoons

garlic crusher

wooden spoon

measuring jug

tin opener

chopping board

sharp knife

Instructions

STEP 1

Bring a small saucepan of water to the boil and carefully lower in the eggs using the slotted spoon. Set a timer for 7 mins if you like your eggs a little runny in the middle, or 8 mins for a set yolk. Have a bowl of cold water nearby. When the timer beeps, scoop the eggs from the hot water using your spoon and plunge them into the cold water. Set aside to cool.

STEP 2

Fill a medium saucepan with enough water to come halfway up the side of the pan. Bring the water to the boil over a high heat, reduce the heat, then lower in the noodles and season the water with a pinch of salt. Cook for 5 mins, or until just cooked – test one noodle to see if it's done. Drain the noodles and drizzle over 1 tbsp oil while they're in the colander. Toss the oil through the noodles to prevent them from sticking together.

STEP 3

Peel the garlic cloves and crush them to a paste using a garlic crusher.

STEP 4

Pour the remaining 1 tbsp oil into the medium saucepan (no need to wash it first), and turn the heat to medium. Add the garlic and ginger, stirring for 1 min until sizzling, then add the turmeric and stir for another 30 secs.

STEP 5

Add the stock, coconut milk, soy sauce and sugar to the pan. Bring to a gentle simmer and bubble, for 2 mins.

STEP 6

Cut the sugar snap peas in half on an angle, then drop them into the hot soup and cook for 1 min. Thinly slice the spring onions.

STEP 7

Divide the noodles between four shallow bowls. Use a ladle to spoon over the hot soup and sugar snap peas. Carefully peel the eggs, then cut them in half and serve 2 halves on top of each serving of noodles, before scattering with the spring onions and coriander.

Giant couscous salad with charred veg & tangy pesto

Ingredients

2-3 raw beetroot (320g), peeled and chopped

3 red onions (320g), cut into wedges

2 green or orange peppers, deseeded and cubed

1 tbsp olive oil

320g cherry tomatoes

200g wholewheat giant couscous

For the pesto

7g fresh coriander, roughly chopped

15g flat-leaf parsley, roughly chopped

1 garlic clove

1 green chilli, deseeded

½ tsp cumin

1 tbsp apple cider vinegar

1 tbsp olive oil

40g pine nuts, lightly toasted

Instructions

STEP 1

Heat the oven to 200C/180C fan/gas 6. In a bowl, toss the beetroot, onions and peppers together with the oil, then spread out on a large roasting tray lined with baking paper and roast for 35 mins. Scatter over the cherry tomatoes, then return to the oven for 10 mins more until the tomatoes have softened and the vegetables are tender.

STEP 2

Meanwhile, cook the couscous following pack instructions, then rinse and drain. To make the pesto, put the coriander and half the parsley in a bowl with the garlic, chilli, cumin, vinegar, oil and 25g of the pine nuts. Add 2 tbsp water, then blitz with a hand blender until smooth or use a small food processor.

STEP 3

Toss the roasted veg and chopped parsley through the couscous and pile on the pesto, then scatter with the remaining pine nuts. Serve the salad immediately.

TASTY HIGH FIBRE DINNER RECIPES

Posh egg, chips & beans

Ingredients

4 large baking potatoes, cut into wedges

2 tbsp olive oil

1 onion, finely chopped

1 tsp smoked paprika

1 thyme sprig

400g can chopped tomatoes

2 x 400g cans cannellini beans

4 eggs

handful chopped flat-leaf parsley

Directions

STEP 1

Heat oven to 200C/180C fan/gas 6. Tip the potatoes into a large roasting tin and toss with 1 tbsp of the oil and some seasoning. Bake for 45 mins-1 hr until crisp and golden, tossing them again halfway through.

STEP 2

Meanwhile, heat the remaining oil in a pan. Add the onion and cook for 10-15 mins until starting to soften, then add the paprika, thyme, chopped tomatoes and beans (including the liquid from the can) and stir well. Simmer for 15 mins, or until thickened, then discard the thyme sprig.

STEP 3

Fry or poach the eggs. Serve alongside the wedges and beans and garnish with the parsley.

Lentil & tuna salad

Ingredients

2 tbsp sherry vinegar

1 tsp Dijon mustard

2 garlic cloves, finely grated

50ml olive oil

2 x 250g pouches ready-cooked puy lentils

2 x 160g cans tuna steaks in spring water, drained and flaked

160g cherry tomatoes, halved (about 10)

2 ready-roasted peppers, chopped

handful of parsley, finely chopped

½ small bunch of chives, finely chopped, plus extra to garnish

Directions

STEP 1

Whisk the vinegar, mustard and garlic together in a small bowl. Slowly drizzle in the oil, whisking as you go, until emulsified, then season to taste.

STEP 2

Add the lentils, tuna, tomatoes, peppers and herbs to a large bowl and toss together. Pour over the dressing and toss again. Divide between four bowls and garnish with the remaining chives.

Roasted carrot & whipped feta tart

Ingredients

large bunch of carrots with tops (about 800g)

2 tsp olive oil

1 tsp za'atar

2 tsp honey

125-150ml extra virgin olive oil

2 garlic cloves, roughly chopped

50g walnuts, roughly chopped

40g grated parmesan or vegetarian hard cheese

25g parsley, roughly chopped, plus whole leaves to serve

200g feta drained and crumbled (vegetarian, if needed)

150g Greek yogurt

1 lemon, zested

500g block puff pastry

1 egg, beaten

Directions

STEP 1

Heat the oven to 200C/180C fan/gas 6. Trim off the carrot tops, discarding any tough stems, then set aside. Halve the carrots lengthways, tip into a roasting tin and toss with the olive oil and some seasoning. Roast for 25-30 mins until tender and golden, stirring once or twice to ensure they don't stick. Stir in the za'atar and honey, and set aside.

STEP 2

Meanwhile, tip the reserved carrot tops and extra virgin olive oil into a food processor. Season and blitz, scraping down the sides occasionally until finely chopped. Add the garlic, walnuts, parmesan and parsley, and pulse until combined. Pour in another splash of olive oil, if needed. Transfer to a bowl and season to taste. Clean out the food processor, then tip in the feta, yogurt, most of the lemon zest and some seasoning. Blitz until smooth and creamy.

STEP 3

Put a large baking tray in the oven to heat up. Roll the pastry out on a sheet of baking parchment into a roughly 40 x 30cm rectangle. Gently score a 2cm border around the edge using a sharp knife. Brush the beaten egg all over the pastry and sprinkle a large pinch of sea salt around the border. Carefully slide the pastry onto the hot baking tray using the parchment to help you, and bake for 15-20 mins until golden and puffed up. Remove from the oven and gently press the middle down using the back of a metal spoon. Cool for 5-10 mins, then spread the whipped feta over the middle and arrange the roasted carrots on top. Drizzle over the pesto, scatter over the parsley and the remaining lemon zest, and cut into slices to serve.

Vegan aubergine no-parmigiana

Ingredients

2 tbsp olive oil, plus 2 drops for the baking sheets

3 aubergines, sliced lengthways, about ½cm thick

For the tomato sauce

2 onions, finely chopped

2 garlic cloves, finely grated

800g chopped tomatoes

1 tsp dried oregano

1 tbsp balsamic vinegar

400g can borlotti beans, drained

15g fresh basil leaves, chopped, plus a few for scattering

For the topping

400g can cannellini beans, drained

150ml soya milk

1 tbsp miso paste

30g pine nuts

4 handfuls rocket

Directions

STEP 1

Heat the oven to 200C/180C fan/gas 6. Line two baking sheets with baking parchment, then cover each one lightly with a drop of oil. Press on the aubergine slices, then turn them over so they end up with just a tiny slick of oil on both sides. Roast in the oven for 15-20 mins until tender.

STEP 2

While the aubergines are cooking, make the sauce. Heat the 2 tbsp oil in a pan and fry the onions and garlic over a low heat until softened. Tip in the tomatoes, oregano, balsamic vinegar, borlotti beans and half the basil, then cover and simmer for 15 mins.

STEP 3

To make the topping, put the cannellini beans in a bowl with the soya milk and miso paste, and blitz with a hand blender until smooth.

STEP 4

Cover the base of a large shallow ovenproof dish (about 20cm x 25cm) with half the tomato sauce. Take a third of the aubergine slices, including all of the end pieces – roughly chop the end pieces and arrange over the tomato sauce with the slices. Spread with the rest of the tomato sauce and all of the remaining slices of aubergine to seal in the sauce. Pour over the miso mixture, scatter over the pine nuts, then cover with foil and bake for 40 mins. Uncover then cook for 10 mins more until the topping is set. Scatter with the remaining basil. If you're following the Healthy Diet Plan, serve half now with half the rocket. Chill the rest for another day. Will keep for three days. Reheat in the microwave until piping hot.

Loaded potato skins with speedy baked beans

Ingredients

2 baking potatoes (about 250g each)

drizzle of rapeseed oil

50g mature cheddar, finely grated

2 spring onions, white parts finely chopped (save the greens for another recipe)

For the beans

½ tsp rapeseed oil

2 garlic cloves, finely grated

2 tbsp tomato purée

1 tbsp balsamic vinegar

1 tsp smoked paprika

400g can cannellini beans

Directions

STEP 1

Heat the oven to 220C/200C fan/gas 7. Rub the potatoes with a small drop of the oil, then put on a baking tray and bake for 50 mins until almost tender. Toss the cheese and onion together and set aside.

STEP 2

Meanwhile, make the beans. Heat the rest of the oil in a small non-stick pan and fry the garlic over a low heat for about a minute, stirring to soften. Add the tomato purée, vinegar and paprika, and cook, stirring, for about a minute more. Tip in the beans and the liquid from the can. Cook for a few minutes so the beans are coated in the sauce, then turn off the heat. Set aside until the potatoes are ready.

STEP 3

After the potatoes have had their 50 mins, remove from the oven and halve lengthways. Carefully scoop out the middles using a teaspoon to create a shell, with an even layer of potato all the way round. Don't take out too much, just about 50g from each potato. Pile on the cheese and onion, then return to the oven for 15 mins until golden. To serve, gently reheat the beans and spoon on top of the cheesy potato skins.

Tomato & oregano orzo with beef koftas

Ingredients

500g 20% beef mince

2 tbsp olive oil

1 large onion, finely chopped

6 garlic cloves, thinly sliced

2 tsp paprika

1 heaped tbsp dried oregano

2 tbsp tomato purée

2 x 400g cans chopped tomatoes

300g orzo

50g unsalted butter

1 heaped tsp pul biber

150g Greek yogurt, to serve

Directions

STEP 1

Put the beef in a large bowl, season with salt and pepper and mix in using your hands. Form into balls (you should have about 40, at around 13g each). Set aside.

STEP 2

Heat the oil in a large lidded pan over a medium-high heat and fry the onions until beginning to soften and turn golden, about 5-6 mins. Add the garlic and cook for 2 mins until softened but not browned.

STEP 3

Add the koftas and cook for 6-7 mins until browned all over, being careful not to stir too much as they will break. Instead, gently shake the pan to move them.

STEP 4

Add the paprika, oregano, tomato purée, tomatoes, and 1 tbsp sugar, and season with salt and pepper. Shake the pan to mix and leave to cook for 5-6 mins, then carefully stir in the meatballs (they should be just cooked and firm enough to stir now). Cover and cook for 10 mins.

STEP 5

Remove the lid, scatter in the orzo and pour in 500ml water. Stir well. Cook for 20 mins until the orzo is cooked and has absorbed the liquid.

STEP 6

Melt the butter in a small saucepan over a medium-low heat, add the pul biber and turn off the heat. Allow to infuse for a minute or so, swirling the pan. Serve the orzo and koftas, dolloped with yogurt and the spiced butter poured over.

Moroccan-style vegetable platter

Ingredients

2 tbsp rapeseed oil

2 garlic cloves, finely chopped

2 aubergines (about 500g), sliced

4 tomatoes, cut into wedges

1 tsp ground cumin

10g coriander, chopped

10g parsley, chopped

1 lemon, juiced

8 flatbreads

250g pack cooked beetroot, sliced

2 x 80g packs pomegranate seeds

1 mint sprig (optional)

For the dip

320g frozen baby broad beans

1 tsp cumin seeds

2 large garlic cloves

1 tbsp extra virgin olive oil

1 tsp smoked paprika

Directions

STEP 1

For the dip, boil the broad beans for 7 mins, then drain, reserving the cooking water. Tip into a bowl with the cumin, garlic, oil, paprika and 6 tbsp of the reserved water, then blitz using a hand blender until smooth. Spoon into two small bowls.

STEP 2

Heat the oil in a pan over a medium heat and cook the garlic and aubergines, covered, for 10 mins, stirring occasionally until tender and slightly charred. Add the tomatoes and cumin, and cook for 5-10 mins, then turn off the heat. Add the herbs and lemon juice.

STEP 3

Serve half on a platter with one bowl of dip, four flatbreads and half the beetroot, along with the pomegranate seeds and mint, if using. You can warm the flatbreads in a frying pan or microwave before serving. Chill the remainder to eat cold the next day. Will keep covered and chilled for a day.

TASTY HIGH FIBRE SNACKS RECIPES

Brummie bacon cakes

Ingredients

3 rashers streaky bacon (we used smoked)

225g self-raising flour, plus extra for dusting

25g butter, cold and cut into small pieces

75g mature cheddar, grated

150ml milk, plus 2 tbsp extra for glazing

1 tbsp tomato ketchup

½ tsp Worcestershire sauce

Instructions

STEP 1

Heat grill to high and grill the bacon for 10 mins, turning halfway, until crisp. Cool for a few mins. Meanwhile, heat oven to 180C/160C fan/gas 4 and line a baking sheet with parchment. Sift the flour and ½ tsp salt into a bowl, add the butter, then rub in to the texture of fine breadcrumbs. Cut the bacon into small pieces and add to the bowl with a third of the cheese.

STEP 2

Mix the milk, ketchup and Worcestershire sauce in a jug. Pour into the bacon mixture, stirring briefly, to make a soft dough. Flour the work surface, turn the dough onto it and shape into an 18cm round. Brush with milk, then cut into 8 wedges with a large knife.

STEP 3

Arrange the wedges on the baking sheet and sprinkle with the remaining cheese. Bake for 20-30 mins or until risen and golden brown, and serve warm (or cool on a wire rack, and store in an airtight container). Warm the bacon cakes through in a low oven (140C/120C fan/gas 1) if you've made them in advance.

Microwave butternut squash risotto

Ingredients

250g risotto rice

700ml hot vegetable stock

1 medium butternut squash

big handful grated parmesan (or vegetarian alternative), plus extra

handful sage leaves, roughly chopped

Instructions

STEP 1

Tip the rice into a large bowl, then add 500ml of the hot vegetable stock. Cover with cling film and microwave on High for 5 mins. Meanwhile, peel and cut the squash into medium chunks (see tip, below). Stir the rice, then add the squash and the rest of the stock. Re-cover with cling film, then microwave for another 15 mins, stirring halfway, until almost all the stock is absorbed and the rice and squash are tender.

STEP 2

Leave the risotto to sit for 2 mins, then stir in the parmesan and sage. Serve topped with more grated cheese.

Burmese tofu fritters (tohu jaw)

Ingredients

2 tbsp vegetable oil, plus extra for the dish and fryer

100g gram flour

¼ tsp salt

1 tsp vegetable bouillon powder

¼ tsp ground turmeric

¼ tsp baking powder

For the dipping sauce

1 ½ tbsp golden caster sugar

2 tbsp fish sauce

2 tbsp light soy sauce

2 limes, juiced

2 finger chillies, sliced into rings

3 garlic cloves, crushed

Instructions

STEP 1

Mix all the Ingredients for the dipping sauce in a bowl. Cover and set aside.

STEP 2

Oil a 15 x 20cm casserole dish. Put the flour, salt, bouillon powder, turmeric, baking powder and 350ml water in a large bowl and whisk thoroughly. Cover and leave somewhere cool for 2 hrs, whisking occasionally.

STEP 3

Pour 250ml boiling water into a large saucepan over a high heat. Add the oil, then pour in the flour mixture and stir slowly with a large spoon. Reduce the heat to medium-high. Continue stirring for up to 10 mins until the mixture starts to bubble and forms a thick, custard-like consistency. Pour into the casserole dish and leave at room temperature to set and cool completely.

STEP 4

Drain away any excess liquid, wrap the tofu in kitchen paper and place back in the dish. At this point, you can cover and chill for up to 48 hrs until needed.

STEP 5

When you're ready to fry the fritters, unwrap the tofu and slice it into 5 x 3 x 1cm rectangles.

STEP 6

Heat a wok or deep-fat fryer with 5cm of oil (no more than one-third full) until you can feel waves of heat when you hold your hand 10cm above the fryer. Gently lower 3 or 4 tofu rectangles into the hot oil – they should start to sizzle almost at once. Fry for 3 mins until golden, then flip gently and fry for a further 3 mins. Remove with a slotted spoon and drain in a colander set over a dish to catch excess oil. Repeat with the next batch.

STEP 7

When you've fried all the tofu fritters, tip them back into the hot oil and fry for a further 4-5 mins for extra crispness. Drain the tofu fritters on plenty of kitchen paper and serve with the garlic dipping sauce or a sweet chilli sauce.

Quick tomato risotto

Ingredients

• 250g risotto rice

• 1 onion, finely chopped

- 50g butter

- 250ml vegetable stock

- 500ml carton passata

- 500g punnet cherry tomato

- 100g ball mozzarella, drained and cut into large chunks

- grated parmesan (or vegetarian alternative) and shredded basil, to serve

Directions

- STEP 1

Tip the rice, onion and half the butter into a large microwave-proof bowl. Cover and cook in the microwave on High for 3 mins. Stir in the stock and passata, then continue to cook, uncovered, for 10 mins. Give it a good stir and mix in the tomatoes and mozzarella. Microwave on High for a further 8 mins until the rice is cooked and the tomatoes have softened.

- STEP 2

Leave the risotto to relax for a few mins, then stir in the remaining butter, parmesan and basil. Season to taste and serve straight from the bowl.

Instant frozen berry yogurt

Ingredients

• 250g frozen mixed berry

• 250g Greek yogurt

• 1tbsp honey or agave syrup

Our Most Popular Alternative

Black pepper chicken & lemon yogurt

Directions

• STEP 1

Blend berries, yogurt and honey or agave syrup in a food processor for 20 seconds, until it comes together to a smooth ice-cream texture. Scoop into bowls and serve.

Greek salad omelette

Ingredients

• 10 eggs

• handful of parsley leaves, chopped (optional)

• 2 tbsp olive oil

• 1 large red onion, cut into wedges

• 3 tomatoes, chopped into large chunks

• large handful black olives, (pitted are easier to eat)

• 100g feta cheese, crumbled

Directions

• STEP 1

Heat the grill to high. Whisk the eggs in a large bowl with the chopped parsley, pepper and salt, if you want. Heat the oil in a large non-stick frying pan, then fry the onion wedges over a high heat for about 4 mins until they start to brown around the edges. Throw in the tomatoes and olives and cook for 1-2 mins until the tomatoes begin to soften.

• STEP 2

Turn the heat down to medium and pour in the eggs. Cook the eggs in the pan, stirring them as they begin to set, until half cooked, but still runny in places – about 2 mins. Scatter over the feta, then place the pan under the grill for 5-6 mins until omelette is puffed up and golden. Cut into wedges and serve straight from the pan.

Feta, tomato & olive loaded fries

Ingredients

• 400g frozen French fries

• 1 tsp dried oregano

• 2 tsp olive oil

• ¼ finely chopped cucumber

• 10 pitted and halved black olives

• 6 finely chopped cherry tomatoes

• 1 tbsp finely chopped parsley

• 3 tbsp Greek yogurt

• 40g crumbled feta

Directions

• STEP 1

Toss the French fries with the dried oregano and olive oil, then cook following pack instructions.

• STEP 2

While the fries are cooking, mix the cucumber with the black olives, cherry tomatoes and parsley. Mix the Greek yogurt with half of the crumbled feta in a separate bowl. Tip the fries into a serving dish, top with the salad and yogurt mixture, then scatter over the remaining crumbled feta. Season and serve.

TASTY LOW FAT DIET RECIPES

TASTY LOW FAT BREAKFAST RECIPES

Cinnamon porridge with baked bananas

Ingredients

• 80g porridge oats

• 150ml semi-skimmed milk

• ½ tsp ground cinnamon

• 1 large ripe banana (120g), halved lengthways and cut in half

• ½ orange, zested and juiced

• 200g plain bio yogurt

• 2 tsp toasted three-seed mix

Directions

- STEP 1

Put the oats, milk, 450ml water and cinnamon in a pan. Bring to the boil, then turn the heat to low, stirring often, for 5 mins until thickened.

- STEP 2

Meanwhile, put the bananas in a dish with the orange zest and juice. Cover and microwave on high for 1½-2 mins until softened. Tip the porridge into bowls and top with the yogurt, banana and seeds.

Smoothie bowl

Ingredients

- 200g frozen mixed berries

- 1 ripe banana

- 75ml oat milk

- 1 tsp maple syrup

- ½ tbsp vanilla protein powder, vegan version if needed

To top

• sliced kiwis, bananas and fresh berries

• 25g granola

• 1 tbsp mixed nuts and seeds

• 1 tbsp almond butter

Directions

• STEP 1

Put the berries, banana, oat milk, maple syrup and protein powder in a powerful blender and blend until smooth. Add a splash more milk if needed, but remember it needs to be quite thick.

• STEP 2

Spoon the smoothie into a bowl and dot over the fresh fruit, granola and mixed nuts and seeds. Drizzle over the almond butter to serve.

Breakfast peppers & chickpeas with tofu

Ingredients

- 1-2 tbsp olive oil

- 2 onions (320g), halved and thinly sliced

- 1 orange pepper, halved, deseeded and sliced

- 1 red chilli, deseeded and sliced

- 400g can chopped tomatoes

- 2 tbsp tomato purée

- 2 tsp vegetable bouillon powder

- 1 tsp dried oregano

- 1 tsp smoked paprika, plus extra for sprinkling

- 2 x 400g cans chickpeas

- 280g pack extra-firm tofu

- 240g soya yogurt

- 2 garlic cloves, finely grated

- 4 tbsp chopped parsley

Directions

• STEP 1

Heat 1 tbsp oil in a large, deep frying pan over a medium heat. Tip in the onions, cover and cook for 5 mins. Remove the lid and stir the onions – they should have softened and started to brown in places. Stir in the pepper, chilli, chopped tomatoes, tomato purée, bouillon powder, oregano, paprika and chickpeas, along with the liquid from the cans. Cover and simmer for 15-20 mins until slightly thickened.

• STEP 2

Meanwhile, slice half the tofu and fry in ½ tbsp oil over a medium heat until lightly golden. Combine the yogurt and garlic in a small bowl. Serve the tomato and chickpea mixture with the tofu, half the yogurt and a scattering of parsley and extra paprika.

Ultimate Seville orange marmalade

Ingredients

• 1.3kg Seville orange

• 2 lemons, juice only

• 2.6kg preserving or granulated sugar

Directions

• STEP 1

Put the whole oranges and lemon juice in a large preserving pan and cover with 2 litres/4 pints water - if it does not cover the fruit, use a smaller pan. If necessary weight the oranges with a heat-proof plate to keep them submerged. Bring to the boil, cover and simmer very gently for around 2 hours, or until the peel can be easily pierced with a fork.

• STEP 2

Warm half the sugar in a very low oven. Pour off the cooking water from the oranges into a jug and tip the oranges into a bowl. Return cooking liquid to the pan. Allow oranges to cool until they are easy to handle, then cut in half. Scoop out all the pips and pith and add to the reserved orange liquid in the pan. Bring to the boil for 6 minutes, then strain this liquid through a sieve into a bowl and press the pulp through with a wooden spoon - it is high in pectin so gives marmalade a good set.

• STEP 3

Pour half this liquid into a preserving pan. Cut the peel, with a sharp knife, into fine shreds. Add half the peel to the liquid in the preserving pan with the warm sugar. Stir over a low heat until all the sugar has dissolved, for about 10 minutes, then bring to the boil and bubble rapidly for 15- 25 minutes until setting point is reached.

• STEP 4

Take pan off the heat and skim any scum from the surface. (To dissolve any excess scum, drop a small knob of butter on to the surface, and gently stir.) Leave the marmalade to stand in the pan for 20 minutes to cool a little and allow the peel to settle; then pot in sterilised jars, seal and label. Repeat from step 3 for second batch, warming the other half of the sugar first.

Healthy pesto eggs on toast

Ingredients

• 2-4 thin slices rye sourdough (about 70g total, depending on the size of the loaf)

• 2 eggs

• 170g tomatoes on-the-vine

• 160g baby spinach

• pinch of chilli flakes (optional)

For the pesto

• 1 garlic clove

• 10g basil

• 1 tbsp pine nuts

• 1 tbsp rapeseed oil

• 1 tbsp finely grated parmesan or vegetarian alternative

Directions

• STEP 1

To make the pesto, peel the garlic clove and put in a small food processor along with the basil, pine nuts, oil and 2 tbsp water. Blitz until smooth, then stir in the cheese. Or, blitz using a hand blender.

• STEP 2

Toast the bread and divide between two plates. Cook the pesto in a frying pan over a medium heat for 30 seconds, stirring. Crack the eggs into one side of the pan, put the tomatoes in the other, and fry in the pesto until the eggs are cooked to your liking.

• STEP 3

Lift out the eggs and put each one on a slice of toast. Add the spinach to the pan with the tomatoes, turn the heat up to high and cook until wilted, about 2-3 mins. The tomatoes should be soft. Spoon the veg onto the other toast slice and sprinkle with the chilli flakes, if you like.

Spinach-Avocado Smoothie

Ingredients

• 1 cup nonfat plain yogurt

• 1 cup fresh spinach

• 1 frozen banana

• ¼ avocado

• 2 tablespoons water

• 1 teaspoon honey

Directions

1. Combine yogurt, spinach, banana, avocado, water and honey in a blender. Puree until smooth.

Cinnamon Streusel Rolls

Ingredients

• 1 cup fat-free milk plus 2 to 3 teaspoons, divided

• 2 teaspoons packed brown sugar

• ¼ cup tub-style 60-70% vegetable oil spread, divided

• 1 teaspoon salt

• ¼ cup warm water (110 to 115 degrees F)

• 1 package active dry yeast

• ¼ cup refrigerated or frozen egg product, thawed, or 1 egg, lightly beaten

• 4-4 1/2 cups all-purpose flour

• ½ cup rolled oats, toasted

• 2 teaspoons ground cinnamon

• ¼ cup chopped pecans, toasted

• ⅓ cup light sour cream

• ¼ cup powdered sugar

• ¼ teaspoon vanilla extract

Directions

1. Heat and stir 1 cup milk, the brown sugar, 2 tablespoons vegetable oil spread, and the salt in a small saucepan just until warm (110 to 115 degrees F); set aside. Combine the warm water and yeast in a large bowl; let stand for 10 minutes. Add egg and the milk mixture to the yeast mixture. Stir in the flour substitute (if using; see Tip) and as much of the remaining all-purpose flour as you can with a wooden spoon.

2. Turn out dough onto a lightly floured surface. Knead in enough of the remaining flour to make a moderately soft dough that is smooth and elastic (3 to 5 minutes total). Shape the dough into a ball. Place in a lightly greased bowl, turning once to grease the surface. Cover and let rise in a warm place until double in size (about 1 hour). Punch down the dough. Turn out onto a lightly floured surface. Cover; let rest for 10 minutes.

3. Meanwhile, lightly grease a 13x9-inch baking pan; set aside. Combine oats and cinnamon in a medium bowl. Using your fingers, blend in the remaining 2 tablespoons vegetable oil spread until the mixture is crumbly. Stir in pecans.

4. Roll the dough into a 15x8-inch rectangle. Sprinkle with the pecan mixture, leaving a 1-inch space along one of the long sides. Starting from the long side with topping, roll up into a spiral. Pinch the dough to seal seam; slice into 15 equal pieces. Arrange the pieces, cut sides up, in the prepared baking pan. Cover and let rise in a warm place until nearly double in size (about 30 minutes).

5. Preheat oven to 375 degrees F. Bake for 25 to 30 minutes or until golden. Cool in the pan on a wire rack for 5 minutes.

6. Meanwhile, combine sour cream, powdered sugar, vanilla, and enough of the remaining 2 to 3 teaspoons milk to make drizzling consistency. Remove the rolls from the pan. Drizzle with icing. Serve warm.

Tips

Tips: If using a sugar substitute, we recommend Sweet'N Low Brown or Sugar Twin Granulated Brown. Follow package directions to use product amount equivalent to 2 tablespoons brown sugar. Nutrition Per Serving with Substitute: same as below, except 189 cal., 31 g carb., 198 mg sodium.

You may substitute 2 cups of either whole-wheat flour, white whole-wheat flour, whole-wheat pastry flour, or whole-grain oat flour for 2 cups of the all-purpose flour called for in this recipe. Nutrition Per Serving with Flour Substitution: same as below, except 189 cal., 32 g carb., 3 g fiber, 6 g pro. (with whole-wheat flour); 188 cal., 198 mg sodium, 32 g carb., 6 g pro. (with white whole-wheat flour); 194 cal., 198 mg sodium, 32 g carb., 3 g fiber. (with white whole-wheat pastry flour); and 200 cal., 6 g total fat, 198 mg sodium, 31 g carb., 6 g pro. (with whole-grain oat flour).

To toast oats, place oats in a large skillet; heat over medium heat for 4 to 5 minutes or until oats are lightly toasted, stirring frequently.

To toast nuts, spread in a shallow baking pan lined with parchment paper. Bake in a 350 degrees F oven for 5 to 10 minutes or until golden, shaking pan once or twice.

TASTY LOW FAT LUNCH RECIPES

Hot & sour soup

Ingredients

• 2 dried chillies, finely chopped

• 60g Chinese char siu pork or roast pork, cut into matchsticks

• 150g peeled and cooked shrimp or prawns

• 15g wood ear mushrooms, soaked for at least 1 hr and cut into matchsticks

• 60g firm tofu, cut into 1cm cubes

• 60g bamboo shoots, cut into matchsticks

• 60g carrot, cut into matchsticks

• 40g peas

• 1.8l chicken stock

• ½ tsp white pepper

• 4 tbsp tomato ketchup

• 1 tsp tomato purée

• ½ tbsp dark soy sauce

• 1 tbsp light soy sauce

• 6 tbsp rice vinegar

• 2 tsp sugar

• 6 tbsp cornflour, mixed with 12 tbsp water to make a runny paste

• 2 eggs, beaten

• ½ tbsp sesame oil

Instructions

• STEP 1

Put all of the Ingredients in a large wok or saucepan (except the cornflour paste, sesame oil and eggs), plus 1½ tsp salt. Slowly bring to the boil, turn down the heat and simmer for 3 mins. Taste and add a little more vinegar or chillies, if you like.

• STEP 2

Give the cornflour paste a good mix, turn up the heat to medium and slowly add the paste to the soup, stirring throughout until it coats the back of a spoon. Turn off the heat and slowly pour in the beaten egg, stirring as you pour. Add the sesame oil and serve.

Slow-cooker pumpkin soup

Ingredients

• 2 tbsp rapeseed oil

• 3 onions (480g), chopped

• 30g ginger, peeled and chopped

• 3 large garlic cloves, chopped

• 1½-2 tbsp medium curry powder

• 1 tsp ground coriander

• ½ tsp crushed dried chillies (optional)

• 1kg pumpkin or butternut squash (flesh only), cut into cubes

• 1 tbsp vegetable bouillon powder (ensure vegan, if needed)

• 400g can coconut milk

• 180g dried red lentils

• 15g coriander, chopped

Instructions

• STEP 1

Heat the oil in a large pan over a medium heat and fry the onions and ginger for 10 mins, stirring occasionally until softened and starting to colour. Stir in the garlic, curry powder, ground coriander and dried chillies, if using, and cook for 1 min more.

• STEP 2

Tip the mixture into a large slow cooker along with all the remaining Ingredients, except the fresh coriander. Add 2 litres water. Cook for 8 hrs on high, or overnight for 15 hrs on low. Stir well, then blitz using a hand blender until smooth. Ladle into bowls and scatter over the fresh coriander to serve. Once completely cool, the soup will keep chilled in an airtight container for 48 hrs or frozen for up to two months. Reheat in a pan over a low heat or in the microwave until piping hot.

Healthy pesto eggs on toast

Ingredients

• 2-4 thin slices rye sourdough (about 70g total, depending on the size of the loaf)

• 2 eggs

• 170g tomatoes on-the-vine

• 160g baby spinach

• pinch of chilli flakes (optional)

For the pesto

• 1 garlic clove

• 10g basil

• 1 tbsp pine nuts

• 1 tbsp rapeseed oil

• 1 tbsp finely grated parmesan or vegetarian alternative

Instructions

• STEP 1

To make the pesto, peel the garlic clove and put in a small food processor along with the basil, pine nuts, oil and 2 tbsp water. Blitz until smooth, then stir in the cheese. Or, blitz using a hand blender.

• STEP 2

Toast the bread and divide between two plates. Cook the pesto in a frying pan over a medium heat for 30 seconds, stirring. Crack the eggs into one side of the pan, put the tomatoes in the other, and fry in the pesto until the eggs are cooked to your liking.

• STEP 3

Lift out the eggs and put each one on a slice of toast. Add the spinach to the pan with the tomatoes, turn the heat up to high and cook until wilted, about 2-3 mins. The tomatoes should be soft. Spoon the veg onto the other toast slice and sprinkle with the chilli flakes, if you like.

Miso lentil & cabbage soup

Ingredients

- 1 tbsp olive oil

- 150g pancetta or chopped bacon

- 300g sliced mushrooms

- 1 tbsp olive oil

- 1 chopped onion

- 4 chopped garlic cloves

- 4 unpeeled sliced carrots

- 3 sliced sticks of celery

- 2 tbsp miso

- 500ml vegetable stock

- 200g washed and drained dried green lentils

- ½ head of chopped white cabbage

- spoonful of thick yogurt

Instructions

- STEP 1

Heat the olive oil in a deep pan over a medium-high heat. You can make this completely veggie, but if you have around 150g pancetta or chopped bacon to use, tip this in and brown all over before removing with a slotted spoon. Stir in the sliced mushrooms and brown all over before transferring to a bowl.

- STEP 2

Pour in the olive oil, then tip in the chopped onion, the garlic cloves, sliced carrots and sticks of celery, leaves and all. Cook gently for 10 mins, until lightly softened. Stir in the miso, preferably red or brown, vegetable stock and 1 litre water and bring to a simmer.

- STEP 3

Finally, stir in the washed and drained dried green lentils and head of chopped white cabbage. Tip the bacon and mushrooms back in. Cover and simmer gently for 30-35 mins until the lentils are tender. Season well and serve with a spoonful of thick yogurt.

Orzo & chickpea soup

Ingredients

- 2 tbsp olive oil

- 1 onion, chopped

- 2 carrots, chopped

- 2 celery sticks, chopped

- 2 tbsp tomato purée

- 3 garlic cloves, chopped

- 3 rosemary or thyme sprigs

- 1 litre vegetable stock

- 400g can chopped tomatoes

- 400g can chickpeas

- parmesan rind or vegetarian alternative (optional)

- 150g orzo

- extra virgin olive oil, to serve

Instructions

• STEP 1

Heat the olive oil in a deep pan over a medium-high heat and cook the onion, carrots and celery, including any leaves for 15 mins until softened. Stir in the tomato purée, garlic cloves and rosemary or thyme sprigs. Cook for a few minutes until the purée is caramelised. Pour in the stock, chopped tomatoes, chickpeas (and the liquid from the can) and parmesan rind, if you have one. Simmer 15 mins.

• STEP 2

Pour boiling water over the orzo in a heatproof bowl and set aside for 15 mins. Drain the orzo, add to the pan and cook for 5-8 mins until the orzo is tender. Fish out and discard the rosemary stalks and cheese rind, then season well. Drizzle over extra virgin olive oil and grated cheese to serve.

Healthy fish pie

Ingredients

• 500g floury potato, cut into chunks

• 1medium swede (weighing about 600g/1lb 5oz), cut into chunks

• 200g tub low-fat soft cheese with garlic and herbs

• 150ml vegetable stock,(we used low sodium stock)

• 4 tsp cornflour, blended with 2 tbsp cold water

• 650g skinless, boneless cod, cut into large chunks

• 100g cooked peeled prawn

• 1 tsp chopped fresh parsley

Instructions

• STEP 1

Cook the potatoes and swede in boiling water until tender (about 20 minutes).

• STEP 2

Preheat the oven to 190C/gas 5/fan 170C.While the potatoes and swede cook, put the soft cheese and stock into a large saucepan and heat gently, stirring with a wooden spoon, until blended and smooth. Now add the blended cornflour and cook until thick.

• STEP 3

Stir the fish into the sauce with the prawns and parsley. Season with some pepper.

• STEP 4

Tip the mixture into a 1.5 litre/2¾ pint baking dish. Drain the potatoes and swede, mash them well and season with black pepper. Spoon the mash over the fish to cover it completely. Bake for 25-30 minutes until piping hot, then transfer to a hot grill for a few minutes to brown the top. Serve with frozen peas or sweetcorn.

Crunchy lettuce salad wraps with sweet satay dip

Ingredients

• 2 Little Gem lettuces, outer leaves only, or loose-leaf lettuce

• 1 cooked chicken breast, chopped

• 1 carrot, grated

• ¼ cucumber, sliced

• 2 radishes, thinly sliced

• handful of coriander or mint leaves

For the sweet satay dip

• 2 tbsp peanut or almond butter

• 1 tbsp sweet chilli sauce

• ½ tsp soy sauce

• 1 lime, ½ juiced, ½ cut into wedges to serve

Instructions

• STEP 1

For the dip, combine the peanut butter, chilli sauce, soy sauce and lime juice in a bowl, loosening with a splash of cold water, if needed, so it's a drizzling consistency.

• STEP 2

Lay a couple of lettuce leaves on a plate and pile a little chicken and some of the veg on each piece. Scatter over the coriander or mint leaves, and squeeze over some lime juice. Drizzle over some of the satay dip, then roll the lettuce around the filling. Serve with the remaining satay on the side for dipping, if you like and the lime wedges for squeezing over.

TASTY LOW FAT DINNER RECIPES

Bloody mary mussels

Ingredients

- 1 tbsp olive oil

- 2 celery sticks, finely chopped

- 1 red chilli, finely chopped

- 1 onion, finely chopped

- 1 lemon, zest peeled into strips, juiced

- 75ml vodka

- 250ml tomato juice

- 5g dashi powder (see tip, below)

- ½ tsp celery salt

- 2 tsp Worcestershire sauce

- a few dashes of hot sauce

- 1tsp sherry vinegar

• ground white pepper, for seasoning

• 2kg mussels, debearded and cleaned

• small handful of parsley, finely chopped

• garlic bread or fries, to serve

Instructions

• STEP 1

Heat the oil in a large, deep saucepan over a medium heat and fry the celery, chilli, onion and lemon zest strips for 8-10 mins until slightly softened, but not coloured. Pour in the vodka, tomato juice, dashi powder, celery salt, Worcestershire sauce, hot sauce, sherry vinegar and 150ml water. Bring to a gentle simmer and bubble for a few minutes until slightly thickened. Season well with white pepper and a dash more hot sauce and Worcestershire sauce, if you like.

• STEP 2

Turn the heat up to high and tip in the cleaned mussels. Put a lid on and steam for 3-4 mins, giving the pan a few vigorous shakes to cook evenly. The shells should be open when cooked; discard any unopened mussels. Sprinkle over

the parsley and serve with garlic bread or fries for mopping
up the sauce.

Sloppy joes with brussels sprout slaw

Ingredients

- 1 tbsp vegetable oil

- 300g lean beef mince

- 1 onion, finely chopped

- 1 green pepper, diced

- 3 garlic cloves, crushed

- 1 tsp ground cumin

- 400ml passata

- 1 tbsp Worcestershire sauce

- 2 tbsp cider vinegar

- 3 tbsp low-fat natural yogurt

- 2 carrots

- 250g brussels sprouts

- 4 wholemeal bread rolls, toasted

Instructions

- STEP 1

Heat the oil in a frying pan and tip in the beef. Brown all over before reducing the heat and adding onion, pepper, garlic and cumin. Cook for 2 mins until fragrant, then add the passata, Worcestershire sauce, half of the vinegar and a pinch of sugar. Simmer gently for 15-20 mins.

- STEP 2

Trim the carrots and, using the grater attachment on a food processor, push through the carrots and sprouts, or finely slice. Combine the remaining vinegar and yogurt in a bowl, and season. Stir in the carrots and sprouts and toss to coat. Season the sloppy joe mixture and serve in toasted buns with the slaw.

Braised shiitake mushrooms & pak choi

Ingredients

* 60g dried whole shiitake mushrooms

* 500g pak choi

* 2 ½ tsp vegetable oil

* 5cm piece ginger, cut into thin matchsticks

* 1 large garlic clove, thinly sliced

* 1 tbsp shaosing wine

* 1 ½ tbsp light soy sauce

* ½ tbsp dark soy sauce

* ½ tbsp sugar

* 1 tbsp oyster sauce

Instructions

* STEP 1

Tip the mushrooms into a bowl and pour over boiling water to submerge them (around 350ml should be enough). Cover, then set aside for 1 hr until rehydrated.

* STEP 2

Thoroughly wash, cut and quarter the pak choi, then set aside. Drain the mushrooms, reserving 300ml of the water, then cut off the stems and evenly slice the stems and mushroom caps into strips.

• STEP 3

Heat 1½ tsp of the vegetable oil in a large frying pan over a medium heat. Fry the ginger and garlic for 1-2 mins until softened, then add the mushroom pieces and cook on a medium-high heat for 1 min. Stir in the shaosing wine, then remove from the heat and set aside.

• STEP 4

Combine the reserved mushroom water with 200ml cold water, tip into a saucepan and bring to the boil over a high heat, then add the mushroom mixture. Tip in the light soy sauce, dark soy sauce, sugar and oyster sauce and mix well. Reduce the heat to medium-low and braise for 15-20 mins until it reduces a little.

• STEP 5

Bring a pan of salted water to the boil over a high heat, add the remaining 1 tsp vegetable oil, then add the pak choi.

Cook for 5-8 mins on a medium heat until the core is tender, then drain. Put the pak choi with the green leaves facing the middle until it forms a flower shape. Lay the braised mushrooms on top and drizzle the mushroom sauce over the mushrooms and pak choi.

Easy lemon chicken

Ingredients

• 2 chicken breasts (around 400g each)

• ½ tbsp cornflour

• ½ tsp white pepper

• 950ml vegetable oil

For the batter

• 2 eggs

• 150g plain flour

• 75g cornflour

• 1 tsp garlic salt or 1/2 tsp each of salt and garlic powder

- 2 tsp garlic powder

- ½ tsp bicarbonate of soda

- 1 tsp Chinese red pepper powder

For the lemon sauce

- 2 lemons, juiced (around 100ml)

- 2 tbsp sugar

- 1½ tsp honey

- 1 tsp cornflour

Instructions

- STEP 1

Slice the chicken breasts horizontally into two thin halves, then sprinkle over the cornflour, ½ tsp salt, the white pepper and ½ tbsp water, then leave to marinate for 20 mins.

- STEP 2

Meanwhile, make the batter. Whisk the eggs in a bowl, then set aside. In a second bowl, combine the plain flour, cornflour, garlic salt, garlic powder, bicarbonate of soda and red pepper powder, then tip half of the mixture into another bowl. Set one aside. Stir the whisked eggs into one bowl of the flour mixture with 3-5 tbsp cold water, adding 1 tbsp at a time. Mix well until it's the consistency of double cream.

• STEP 3

Coat one chicken breast in the batter until evenly covered, then coat in the flour mixture. Rub in the flour using your hands to ensure it's completely coated. Repeat until all four halves of the chicken breasts have been coated.

• STEP 4

Pour the vegetable oil into a medium saucepan (it should be no more than a third full) and heat over a medium-high heat until the oil reaches 160C or forms bubbles around a chopstick. Reduce the heat to medium and slowly lower the chicken breasts into the oil, in batches if your saucepan isn't big enough to do them all at once, then fry for 5 mins, turning over halfway, until pale golden.

• STEP 5

Let the chicken rest for 5 mins and heat the oil on high to 200C, then fry the chicken again for 30 seconds until it forms a deep golden crispy coating. Set aside to cool before cutting into even slices.

• STEP 6

To make the sauce, combine the lemon juice, sugar and honey in a bowl. In a separate bowl, combine the cornflour with 1½ tsp water. Put a pan on a medium heat, tip in the lemon mixture and, once it starts to bubble, slowly add the cornflour mixture until it reaches your desired sauce consistency. Remove from the heat and serve drizzled over the chicken, or as a dipping sauce.

Crunchy lettuce salad wraps with sweet satay dip

Ingredients

• 2 Little Gem lettuces, outer leaves only, or loose-leaf lettuce

• 1 cooked chicken breast, chopped

• 1 carrot, grated

• ¼ cucumber, sliced

* 2 radishes, thinly sliced

* handful of coriander or mint leaves

For the sweet satay dip

* 2 tbsp peanut or almond butter

* 1 tbsp sweet chilli sauce

* ½ tsp soy sauce

* 1 lime, ½ juiced, ½ cut into wedges to serve

Instructions

* STEP 1

For the dip, combine the peanut butter, chilli sauce, soy sauce and lime juice in a bowl, loosening with a splash of cold water, if needed, so it's a drizzling consistency.

* STEP 2

Lay a couple of lettuce leaves on a plate and pile a little chicken and some of the veg on each piece. Scatter over the coriander or mint leaves, and squeeze over some lime juice. Drizzle over some of the satay dip, then roll the lettuce around the filling. Serve with the remaining satay on the side for dipping, if you like and the lime wedges for squeezing over.

Tamarind prawn curry

Ingredients

- 1tbsp vegetable oil

- 1 onion, chopped

- 1 red chilli, finely chopped

- garlic cloves, crushed

- 1tbsp ginger

- 1tsp turmeric

- 1tsp cumin seeds

- 1tsp ground coriander

- 400g cherry tomatoes

- 1tbsp tamarind paste (see tip, below)

- 250g raw king prawns

• 250g cooked basmati rice

• Handful of coriander leaves, to serve

Instructions

• STEP 1

Heat the oil in a frying pan over a medium heat and cook the onion for 5-8 mins until light golden. Stir in the chilli, garlic and ginger, and fry for another minute before adding the spices. Tip in the cherry tomatoes, swirl the can out with a splash of water and stir that into the pan as well.

• STEP 2

Simmer for 5 mins until the tomatoes burst and the sauce thickens. Stir in the tamarind and prawns, and simmer for 2-3 mins until the prawns are cooked. Serve the curry on top of the rice, with the coriander scattered over.

Slow-cooker chicken curry

Ingredients

• 1 large onion, roughly chopped

* 3 tbsp mild curry paste

* 400g can chopped tomatoes

* 2 tsp vegetable bouillon powder

* 1 tbsp finely chopped ginger

* 1 yellow pepper, deseeded and chopped

* 2 skinless chicken legs, fat removed

* 30g pack fresh coriander, leaves chopped

* cooked brown rice, to serve

Instructions

* STEP 1

Put 1 roughly chopped large onion, 3 tbsp mild curry paste, a 400g can chopped tomatoes, 2 tsp vegetable bouillon powder, 1 tbsp finely chopped ginger and 1 chopped yellow pepper into the slow cooker pot with a third of a can of water and stir well.

* STEP 2

Add 2 skinless chicken legs, fat removed, and push them under all the other Ingredients so that they are completely submerged. Cover with the lid and chill in the fridge overnight.

• STEP 3

The next day, cook on Low for 6 hrs until the chicken and vegetables are really tender.

• STEP 4

Stir in the the chopped leaves of 30g coriander just before serving over brown rice.

TASTY LOW FAT SIDE DISH RECIPES

Ratatouille

Ingredients

- 2 large aubergines

- 4 small courgettes

- 2 red or yellow peppers

- 4 large ripe tomatoes

- 5 tbsp olive oil

- supermarket pack or small bunch basil

- 1 medium onion, peeled and thinly sliced

- 3 garlic cloves, peeled and crushed

- 1 tbsp red wine vinegar

- 1 tsp sugar (any kind)

Directions

- STEP 1

Cut 2 large aubergines in half lengthways. Place them on the board, cut side down, slice in half lengthways again and then across into 1.5cm chunks. Cut the ends off 4 small courgettes, then across into 1.5cm slices.

• STEP 2

Peel 2 red or yellow peppers from stalk to bottom. Hold upright, cut around the stalk, then cut into 3 pieces. Cut away any membrane, then chop into bite-size chunks.

• STEP 3

Score a small cross on the base of each of 4 large ripe tomatoes, then put them into a heatproof bowl. Pour boiling water over, leave for 20 secs, then remove. Pour the water away, replace the tomatoes and cover with cold water. Leave to cool, then peel the skin away.

• STEP 4

Quarter the tomatoes, scrape away the seeds with a spoon, then roughly chop the flesh.

• STEP 5

Set a sauté pan over medium heat and when hot, pour in 2 tbsp olive oil. Brown the aubergines for 5 mins on each side until the pieces are soft. Set them aside.

• STEP 6

Fry the courgettes in another tbsp oil for 5 mins, until golden on both sides. Repeat with the peppers. Don't overcook the vegetables at this stage.

• STEP 7

Tear up the leaves from the bunch of basil and set aside. Cook 1 thinly sliced medium onion in the pan for 5 minutes. Add 3 crushed garlic cloves and fry for a further minute. Stir in 1 tbsp red wine vinegar and 1 tsp sugar, then tip in the tomatoes and half the basil.

• STEP 8

Return the vegetables to the pan with some salt and pepper and cook for 5 mins. Serve with basil.

Smoky chickpea salad

Ingredients

* 1 tbsp sunflower oil

* 2 x 400g can chickpeas, drained and rinsed

* 200g carrots, peeled into ribbons or grated

* 200g spinach

* 1 small head of broccoli, roughly chopped

For the dressing

* 2 tsp smoked paprika

* 2 tsp garlic granules

* 2 tsp dried mixed herbs

* 4 tsp maple syrup

* 2 tbsp low-sodium soy sauce

* 4 tsp rice vinegar

* 2 tsp sesame oil

Directions

* STEP 1

Heat the oil in a large pan over a medium heat. Tip in the chickpeas and fry gently for 3-4 mins until sizzling and slightly crispy.

• STEP 2

Whisk together the dressing Ingredients in a bowl, then pour over the chickpeas along with 4 tbsp water and bring to a boil. Cook for 1-2 mins until reduced slightly, remove from the heat, season well and set aside.

• STEP 3

Toss the carrots, spinach and raw broccoli together and divide between plates. Scatter over the chickpeas and a spoonful of the pan juices to dress.

Corn tortillas

Ingredients

• 400g masa harina (corn flour)

Directions

• STEP 1

Put the masa harina in a large bowl, make a well in the middle and add 350g water and ½ tsp salt. Bring together with your hands or a spatula until a dough forms, then knead in the bowl briefly until smooth and well combined. (As there's no gluten in the dough, there's no need to stretch or knead it on your work surface.) If the dough feels sticky, sprinkle over a little more masa, or if it cracks when you fold it, add a splash more water. The more you work the dough, the less gritty it will feel. Cover with a clean tea towel and leave to rest for 10 mins.

• STEP 2

Divide the dough into 20 equal pieces (about 40g each) and roll into balls between your palms. If you have a tortilla press, press each ball between two squares of baking parchment until 2mm thick and 12cm in diameter. Alternatively, roll the dough balls out between two sheets of baking parchment until 2mm thick, then use a 12cm bowl, plate or pastry cutter as a template to cut out the tortillas. Set the tortillas aside and cover with a clean tea towel or sheet of baking parchment to prevent them from drying out while you make the rest. Re-roll any offcuts and press or cut these into tortillas, too.

• STEP 3

Heat a dry, non-stick frying pan over a medium-high heat and fry the tortillas for 1 min until lightly golden and slightly charred in spots. Flip over with a fish slice or tongs and cook on the other side for 1 min more. Wrap in foil, then a tea towel to keep warm while you cook the rest. Will keep, wrapped and in an airtight container in the fridge, for up to two days.

Microwave caraway & pomegranate red cabbage

Ingredients

• 1 red cabbage (around 550g), finely sliced

• 65ml pomegranate juice

• 1 bay leaf

• ½ tsp caraway seeds, lightly crushed

• 2 tsp pomegranate molasses, to serve (optional)

Directions

• STEP 1

Mix everything in a large heatproof bowl, except the pomegranate molasses, and season well.

• STEP 2

Cover and cook on high for 10 mins. Stir, then cook for 10 mins more. Drizzle with the molasses, if you like. Will keep chilled for up to three days. Leave to cool first.

Braised shiitake mushrooms & pak choi

Ingredients

• 60g dried whole shiitake mushrooms

• 500g pak choi

• 2 ½ tsp vegetable oil

• 5cm piece ginger, cut into thin matchsticks

• 1 large garlic clove, thinly sliced

• 1 tbsp shaosing wine

• 1 ½ tbsp light soy sauce

• ½ tbsp dark soy sauce

• ½ tbsp sugar

• 1 tbsp oyster sauce

Directions

• STEP 1

Tip the mushrooms into a bowl and pour over boiling water to submerge them (around 350ml should be enough). Cover, then set aside for 1 hr until rehydrated.

• STEP 2

Thoroughly wash, cut and quarter the pak choi, then set aside. Drain the mushrooms, reserving 300ml of the water, then cut off the stems and evenly slice the stems and mushroom caps into strips.

• STEP 3

Heat 1½ tsp of the vegetable oil in a large frying pan over a medium heat. Fry the ginger and garlic for 1-2 mins until softened, then add the mushroom pieces and cook on a medium-high heat for 1 min. Stir in the shaosing wine, then remove from the heat and set aside.

• STEP 4

Combine the reserved mushroom water with 200ml cold water, tip into a saucepan and bring to the boil over a high heat, then add the mushroom mixture. Tip in the light soy sauce, dark soy sauce, sugar and oyster sauce and mix well. Reduce the heat to medium-low and braise for 15-20 mins until it reduces a little.

• STEP 5

Bring a pan of salted water to the boil over a high heat, add the remaining 1 tsp vegetable oil, then add the pak choi. Cook for 5-8 mins on a medium heat until the core is tender, then drain. Put the pak choi with the green leaves facing the middle until it forms a flower shape. Lay the braised mushrooms on top and drizzle the mushroom sauce over the mushrooms and pak choi.

Mango & green bean salad with honey & passion fruit dressing

Ingredients

• 200g fine green beans, trimmed

• 3 passion fruits

• 1-2 tbsp honey

• 2 tbsp extra virgin olive oil

• 10g ginger, peeled and finely grated

• ½ -1 red chilli deseeded and finely chopped, depending on how much heat you prefer

• squeeze of lime juice, to taste

• 1kg mangoes

• 1 tbsp chopped coriander

• 1 tbsp mint leaves

Directions

• STEP 1

Bring a large pan of salted water to the boil over a high heat and cook the green beans for 2 mins until just tender. Drain and rinse under cold running water to halt the cooking process and retain the vibrant colour. Pat dry with kitchen paper and set aside.

• STEP 2

Halve the passion fruits, scoop the pulp into a small pan and bring to a simmer over a low heat. Cook for 5 mins until the pulp has thickened enough to coat the back of a spoon. Remove from the heat and press the pulp through a sieve into a small bowl, discarding the seeds.

• STEP 3

Whisk 1 tbsp honey into the passion fruit purée, followed by the oil, ginger, chilli and lime juice. Season and taste – you might need to add a little more honey or lime juice. Aim for a balance of sweet, tart and acidic.

• STEP 4

Slice down through the mangoes along both sides of the stone so you end up with two 'cheeks'. Using a tablespoon, scoop the flesh from the skin and cut into 3cm chunks. Scrape and roughly chop any fleshy bits from the stones.

• STEP 5

Transfer the mango flesh to a shallow serving dish, drizzle with 3 tbsp of the dressing, then gently spoon over the green beans. Stir the coriander into the remaining dressing and pour it over the beans, then scatter with mint and serve.

Soy & sesame glazed celeriac

Ingredients

- 1½kg celeriac, peeled

- 1 tbsp gochujang

- 2 tbsp soy sauce

- 1 tbsp honey

- 1 tbsp rice vinegar

- 1 tbsp sesame oil

- ½ tbsp sesame seeds

- 3 spring onions, finely sliced

- cooked white rice, to serve

Directions

- STEP 1

Heat the oven to 200/180C fan/gas 6. Cut the celeriac into 2-3cm wedges and put in a roasting tin.

- STEP 2

Whisk the gochujang, soy, honey, vinegar, sesame oil and sesame seeds together until smooth and emulsified. Pour over the celeriac and, using your hands, toss to coat. Roast for 20 mins. Turn, then cook for a further 15 mins. Turn again and cook for a final 5 mins until sticky and caramelised, and the celeriac is tender. Serve with the spring onions scattered over alongside cooked rice, with any leftover glaze on the side.

PART V: FINALLY

To follow a low-fat diet plan, you choose foods that contain less fat or consume smaller portions of fatty foods. Usually, foods are not explicitly forbidden, but to stay compliant with the plan, you might have to eat a smaller-than-usual portion of foods that are higher in fat. For instance, chocolate lovers can still consume their favorite food, but they only consume an amount that keeps them within their fat intake goals.

On a low-fat diet, you choose foods based on fat content. Foods that are low in fat are often foods that are also low in calories, but not always. In many processed foods, fat is replaced by starch, sugar, or other ingredients that still contribute calories.

For example, some low-fat salad dressings replace oil with sugar or thickeners that reduce the fat content but increase sugar and sometimes calorie content. Some fat-free coffee creamers contain oil just like their full-fat counterparts, but the fat contained in a single serving is minimal enough that the food is allowed to be labeled as fat-free.

Natural low-fat or fat-free foods in their whole form (that is, not heavily processed) are more likely to be more nutrient-dense. For example, many fruits and vegetables are naturally low in calories and fat. If weight loss is your goal, these foods help you feel full without feeling like you're on a diet.

Some popular low-fat diets, however, reduce fat intake more substantially. The Ornish diet, for example, recommends consuming no more than 10% of your calories from fat and suggests that those calories should only come from "fat that occurs naturally in grains, vegetables, fruit, beans, legumes, soy foods—and small amounts of nuts & seeds."

Calculate Your Fat Intake

Low-fat diets usually require you to count macronutrients and/or calories. So, if your goal is to stay under 30% of daily calories from fat, you'll need to calculate your total calorie intake and make sure that your fat grams don't contribute more than 30%.

Total Grams of Fat Per Day = (Total Calories Per Day x 0.3) / 9 Calories Per Gram of Fat

• If you consume 2000 calories per day, 600 calories can come from fat on a low-fat diet. Since each gram of fat contains 9 calories, you would be able to consume about 66.7 grams of fat per day.

• Those consuming 1800 calories per day would be able to consume 540 calories from fat, or 60 grams.

• Those consuming 1500 calories per day could consume 450 calories from fat or 50 grams of fat.

Read Labels and Count Grams

If you are new to counting calories or tracking macros, you may find that using a smartphone app is helpful. Apps like MyFitnessPal or LoseIt! have databases of thousands of food items. You can either scan a product barcode or manually input a specific portion of food to instantly see how many calories and fat grams the food provides.

You can also use a simple food journal to keep track of your fat and nutrition intake. Use the nutrition facts label on the foods you consume (or data from the U.S. Department of Agriculture (USDA) to calculate your fat intake. You'll see that fat is the first listing under calories on the label. In addition to total fat grams, the label is also likely to provide information about saturated fat grams and trans fat grams.

Learn About Different Types of Fat

Most low-fat diets do not make a distinction between different types of fat. If you want to follow a healthy variation of a low-fat diet, you'll want to understand the different types and choose those fatty foods that provide health benefits—specifically monounsaturated and polyunsaturated fats.

Since low-fat diets first became popular, scientists and nutrition experts have learned more about fat and its effects on the body. Monounsaturated fats (found in olives, nuts, and avocados) and polyunsaturated fats (found in fatty fish, walnuts, and seeds) are considered "good fats" because they provide important nutrients and can help reduce cholesterol levels in your blood, lowering your risk of heart disease and stroke.

On the other hand, saturated fat and trans fats (which are being eliminated from processed foods) are known to have negative effects on heart health. According to the American Heart Association, eating foods that contain saturated fats raises the level of cholesterol in your blood, which can increase your risk of heart disease and stroke. Even though the USDA recommends limiting saturated fat to 10% or less of daily calories, the AHA suggests that you limit your saturated fat intake to 5% to 6% of total calories.

5 Tips for Low-Fat Cooking

1. Trim all visible fat and remove the skin from poultry.

2. Refrigerate soups, gravies, and stews, and remove the hardened fat on top before eating.

3. Bake, broil, or grill meats on a rack that allows fat to drip from the meat. Don't fry foods.

4. Sprinkle lemon juice, herbs, and spices on cooked vegetables instead of using cheese, butter, or cream-based sauces.

5. Try plain, nonfat or low-fat yogurt and chives on baked potatoes rather than sour cream. Reduced-fat sour cream still has fat, so limit the amount you use.

When You're Eating Out

Choose simply prepared foods such as broiled, roasted, or baked fish or chicken. Avoid fried or sautéed foods, casseroles, and foods with heavy sauces or gravies.

Ask that your food be cooked without added butter, margarine, gravy, or sauce.

If you're ordering salad, ask for low-fat dressing on the side.

Select fruit, angel food cake, nonfat frozen yogurt, sherbet, or sorbet for dessert instead of ice cream, cake, or pie.

Incorporating a High Fiber Diet into Your Lifestyle

Fiber Supplements: When Are They Necessary?

Doctors often prescribe fiber supplements for the treatment of irritable bowel syndrome (IBS) or constipation. These supplements are considered functional fibers that are isolated from plant sources.

Metamucil (psyllium) is a type of soluble fiber supplement you can use to bulk stool and encourage regular bowel movements.

Dextrin is a type of soluble, prebiotic fiber found in products such as Benefiber that promotes good bacteria for overall digestive health.

Citracel (methylcellulose) and Fibercon (polycarbophil) are other fiber supplement options to keep you regular.

What Happens if You Get Too Much Fiber?

As with everything else in life, too much fiber can be harmful to your health. The U.S. Dietary Guidelines don't specify an upper limit on fiber intake, but it's well known that too much fiber causes gas, bloating, and diarrhea, according to the American Academy of Family Physicians.

A sudden increase in fiber, inadequate fluid intake, and inactivity may also increase the likelihood of these symptoms.

When you consume more than 50 g of fiber per day, you may face a risk of mineral binding, which essentially means your body excretes minerals instead of absorbing them. Some of the minerals at risk of binding with excess fiber intake include calcium and phosphorus, per research in Diabetes

Care. This doesn't mean you should limit fiber; rather, it brings home the importance of ensuring you're consuming enough of the aforementioned minerals.

Tips for Increasing Fiber Intake

You can hit your fiber goal by incorporating fiber-rich foods into your meals and snacks. Here's how:

Make Your Grains Whole

When you're eating a carb, think, How can I make this higher in fiber? One sure bet: Swap out refined white versions for whole grains, suggests the Centers for Disease Control and Prevention (CDC). Choose whole-grain bread over white, brown rice instead of white rice, and whole-wheat pasta over traditional white pasta.

Make-Over Your Snacks

Midday snacks are a great opportunity to sneak in more fiber, such as with sliced, raw veggies, recommends the CDC. Buy them precut (or slice some over the weekend) to have them ready to grab when you need to munch; bring them out while you make dinner to get a few slices in then, too. While you're at it, fold these sliced veggies into wraps and sandwiches, too, for extra crunch.

Rely on Beans

Beans are an excellent source of fiber, and they can be added to a variety of dishes, such as atop a salad and in soups and stews, suggests the Academy of Nutrition and Dietetics. Grab a few of those veggie slices and dip them into bean or hummus dip for a double-dose of fiber.

Sprinkle It On

Flaxseeds and chia seeds are foods that double as fiber supplements — and they're easy to add to oatmeal, in smoothies, and on salads, toast, yogurt, or whatever else you can dream up. One tablespoon of ground flax offers 2 g of fiber, per the USDA. An ounce of chia seeds has a whopping 10 g of fiber.

Opt for Fruit as Dessert

Fruit is nature's candy — and it happens to be packed with fiber. As the CDC recommends, you can fit in extra fiber (as well as vitamins) when you pair a whole fruit with your meal or eat it as dessert. Try a bowl of berries, a ripe, juicy pear, or grab a spoon and dig into a kiwi.